T0210895

Veterinary Epidemiology

Veterinary Epidemiology

An Introduction

Dirk U. Pfeiffer

Tierarzt, Dr.med.vet., PhD, MACVSc, DipECVPH
Veterinary Epidemiology and Public Health Group
The Royal Veterinary College
University of London, UK

WILEY-BLACKWELL

A John Wiley & Sons, Ltd., Publication

This edition first published 2010
© 2010 Dirk U. Pfeiffer

Blackwell Publishing was acquired by John Wiley & Sons in February 2007. Blackwell's publishing programme has been merged with Wiley's global Scientific, Technical, and Medical business to form Wiley-Blackwell.

Registered office
John Wiley & Sons Ltd, The Atrium, Southern Gate, Chichester, West Sussex, PO19 8SQ, United Kingdom

Editorial offices
9600 Garsington Road, Oxford, OX4 2DQ, United Kingdom
2121 State Avenue, Ames, Iowa 50014-8300, USA

For details of our global editorial offices, for customer services and for information about how to apply for permission to reuse the copyright material in this book please see our website at www.wiley.com/wiley-blackwell.

Library of Congress Cataloging-in-Publication Data

Pfeiffer, Dirk, 1958–
    Veterinary epidemiology : an introduction / Dirk U. Pfeiffer.
        p. ; cm.
    Includes bibliographical references and index.
    ISBN 978-1-4051-7694-1 (pbk. : alk. paper) 1. Veterinary epidemiology. I. Title.
    [DNLM: 1. Epidemiologic Methods–veterinary. 2. Animal Diseases–epidemiology.
SF 780.9 P526v 2010]
    SF780.9.P44 2010
    636.089′44–dc22

                                                                    2009035245

A catalogue record for this book is available from the British Library.

Set in 10.5/12.5 pt Sabon by Toppan Best-set Premedia Limited

1   2010

To Susanne, Patrick and my parents.

Contents

Preface

The concept of epidemiology was introduced to me while I was conducting research for my postgraduate Dr.med.vet. thesis in Colombia in 1985, after completing my undergraduate veterinary studies in Germany. Today, veterinary epidemiology is integrated into the undergraduate veterinary course curricula in many countries around the world, recognising its contribution to generating and interpreting the scientific evidence supporting veterinary decision-making. Unfortunately, the vast majority of undergraduate veterinary students still do not recognise the need for a veterinary practitioner to be able to critically evaluate scientific research that informs their diagnostic and therapeutic decisions. Personally, I have found veterinary epidemiology a very exciting field to work in, and that is due to its integrative role between science and decision-making in relation to animal health. It is about collecting data related to real-world problems affecting animals and people, applying theoretical methods to this data for identification of the key relationships in underlying biological systems, and then using that generated knowledge to work towards solving the problems in collaboration with those affected. This basic approach allows veterinary epidemiologists to make contributions to animal and human health in almost any cultural and socio-economic setting around the world.

This book is based on a set of lecture notes which I originally wrote between 1992 and 1999 while teaching epidemiology to undergraduate veterinary students at Massey University, Palmerston North, New Zealand. During this time, the lecture notes were compiled into a book which was made available for free download through the Internet. That digital book has been translated into Thai, Serbian, Japanese and Spanish, and possibly other languages that I am not aware of. It was reviewed and challenged by the large number of postgraduate students that I have taught since 1992, as well as many colleagues who used it around the world. Still, any errors in the previously available digital version and the current book are completely my responsibility. The current book replaces the digital book and is an almost complete rewrite of that version, taking into account new developments and changes in terminology.

The aim of this book is to provide a general introduction to veterinary epidemiology for anyone interested in the subject area, including undergraduate and postgraduate veterinary students, as well as animal health professionals involved in disease control at farm, national or international level. The book is deliberately kept short of detailed examples, so that it allows a quick introduction to most of the important concepts and methods. Suitable references are provided in the text to further information on specific topics, including other veterinary epidemiology textbooks such as the ones by Dohoo *et al.* (2009), Houe *et al.* (2004), Noordhuizen *et al.* (2001), Smith (2006) and Toma *et al.* (1999). The definitions and notation used in the current text are largely consistent with the textbooks by Rothman *et al.* (2008d) and Dohoo *et al.* (2009).

The content of the book is organised using a sequence of steps similar to what one might use during the planning and analysis of epidemiological investigations. Following the introductory chapter, Chapter 2 describes the general concepts of veterinary epidemiology with a particular emphasis on causation. Chapter 3 deals with various methods for quantifying disease risks and rates. Chapter 4 covers the topic of study design, leading on to Chapter 5 which introduces measures of effect. Issues of bias and statistical hypothesis testing are discussed in Chapter 6. Sampling of animal populations is fundamental to good study design and implementation, and this is dealt with in Chapter 7. An area where most veterinarians will have to deal directly with risk and uncertainty is diagnosis; Chapter 8 discusses methods that allow improved interpretation of diagnostic tests. Finally, Chapter 9 is a brief introduction to epidemiological concepts in the context of disease control and eradication.

I hope that this book will fulfil as useful a role as an accessible introductory reference to veterinary epidemiology as did the digital version that used to be freely available via the Internet.

Dirk Pfeiffer

Acknowledgements

I have to thank Ewald Otte who explained the basic concepts of veterinary epidemiology to me in 1985 and then gave me the opportunity to gain practical experience in epidemiological research in his German technical cooperation project in Colombia in 1985. He also introduced me to Roger Morris who mentored me while I was studying with him for a PhD in New Zealand. After I completed my PhD, Roger gave me the opportunity to teach veterinary epidemiology at undergraduate and postgraduate level, resulting in the lecture notes which led to the development of this book.

I also have to thank my postgraduate students and colleagues as well as the participants of the many short courses I have had the privilege to have been involved in as a teacher around the world for reminding me that learning is a lifelong process. They continue to demonstrate to me that my knowledge even about basic epidemiological concepts will always be incomplete.

I also thank Suwicha Kasemsuwan and her colleagues at Kasetsart University in Bangkok who helped to make it possible for me to stay in Thailand so that I finally found the time to finish this book.

I would like to thank the members of our Veterinary Epidemiology and Public Health Group at the Royal Veterinary College for their patience during my five months' absence while writing this book. Katharina Stärk and Javier Guitian were very happy to cover several of my responsibilities while I was on sabbatical. Gilly Kyriacou adapted very quickly to my preference for electronic communication and provided efficient assistance.

I thank Justinia Wood from Wiley Blackwell who convinced me that I should publish this book; she demonstrated a lot of patience during the process. Katy Loftus very competently provided me with editorial support during the production process.

Finally, without my parents encouraging me to work overseas and take on challenges seemingly beyond my perception of my ability, I would never have become an epidemiologist. And I am most grateful to Susanne and Patrick who have always supported my professional ambitions and adventures and even came with me to Bangkok to support me while I was writing this book.

Dirk Pfeiffer

Introduction

Learning objectives

After completing this chapter, you will be able to:

- Describe the relationship between veterinary science, evidence-based veterinary medicine and epidemiology.
- Provide definitions of veterinary epidemiology.

Current and future challenges in animal health and veterinary public health

Over the past 50 years, the veterinary profession has been confronted with a range of challenges relating to animal and public health at the single animal and population level. At the individual animal level, particularly in the context of clinical practice, the importance of probability-based information is now well recognised, and has led to the development of evidence-based veterinary medicine which is discussed briefly below. At the population level, old diseases such as bovine tuberculosis have re-emerged in some settings; previously geographically confined diseases such as bluetongue are expanding their range; and new ones such as bovine spongiform encephalopathy (BSE) have appeared and spread to many countries before being recognised. In parallel, the public develops ever higher expectations with respect to food safety and animal welfare standards. Despite lengthy and very costly disease control campaigns eradication seems to be impossible for some diseases, such as bovine tuberculosis in the United Kingdom or bluetongue infection in Europe.

It is also considered necessary to take into account the economic aspects of disease control at farm or regional level (Rushton 2008). Costly multifactorial disease complexes such as mastitis or cattle lameness have become more common, in some instances associated with more intensive production practices. The latter have also been associated with large-scale disease outbreaks with significant economic and welfare consequences, e.g. with classical swine fever in 1997/98 and avian influenza strain type H7N7 in 2003 in the Netherlands (Stegeman *et al.* 2000, Stegeman *et al.* 2004). The large number of animal movements occurring in the United Kingdom and from there to other European countries was one of the key factors in the extraordinary scale of the foot-and-mouth disease (FMD) outbreak in 2001 (Gibbens and Wilesmith 2002). Worldwide trade in animals and animal-derived products presents new challenges to food safety, as food is being sourced from countries with varying standards of food safety. Climate change as well as increased long-distance movement of livestock and pets is likely to result in changes in the geographical distribution of diseases. New diseases have occurred, such as BSE, which presented a formidable challenge in terms of identification of cause and effective control, while resulting in severe economic consequences for the cattle industry in many countries as well as human fatalities (Wilesmith *et al.* 1991). In recent times, the development of antimicrobial resistance has been recognised as a significant threat to animal and human health, such as in the case of methicillin-resistant *Staphylococcus aureus* (MRSA). Globalisation of human travel allows infectious diseases to spread very quickly around the world as was demonstrated during the outbreak of severe acute respiratory syndrome (SARS) in 2002/3 (Anderson *et al.* 2004). To be able to deal with the above-mentioned challenges as effectively as possible, animal health and welfare policy decision-makers often demand scientific advice that is relevant for immediate to short-term application in animal populations. It has also become evident that the historical separation of surveillance and disease investigation between animals and humans ignores the inherent connectedness of biological systems, and that therefore a so-called 'one medicine' or 'one health' approach is required (Zinsstag *et al.* 2005).

At the individual animal level, veterinarians working in clinical practice have to make a wide range of decisions which depend on probability-based information. Examples are how likely it is that a patient has a certain disease given a particular diagnostic test result, or how likely it is that a specific treatment will result in cure. The answer to these questions requires an understanding of the scientific evidence describing the performance of the diagnostic test or the treatment method used. It is not sufficient to only rely on sources such as textbooks, since they are often out of date, and relying on a single expert's recommendations may result in biased information. Furthermore, the volume of information available in the peer-reviewed literature or through the Internet is often overwhelming and its validity is difficult to determine. Continuing professional development (CPD) activities are essential for veterinarians to keep their knowledge base up to date, but this can be very time-consuming and is unlikely to address the complete spectrum of clinical cases that has to be dealt with in day-to-day practice. Given these constraints, the veterinarian has to aim for an optimum balance between their applied clinical skills and theoretical knowledge, where the former is likely to improve with experience and the latter is likely to decline with time, particularly without effective CPD. Recognising these constraints, evidence-based veterinary medicine (EBVM) has been introduced since the beginning of the 21st century, based on a concept developed a decade earlier in medical science (Cockcroft and Holmes 2003).

Veterinary epidemiology

The challenges to animal and public health mentioned above have in common that they require identification, quantification and intensive examination of multiple, directly or indirectly causal, and often interacting, disease determinants. The science of veterinary epidemiology deals with the investigation of these determinants of disease distribution in animal populations. Productivity and welfare of animals may also be outcomes of interest since disease will usually impact on both, and they may indeed often be what stakeholders will have as their primary focus. Veterinary epidemiology involves the application of a structured scientific approach towards integrating data generated by different scientific disciplines and techniques during an investigation of disease. The emphasis is often on providing scientific evidence that is of immediate relevance for decision-making.

In the context of providing epidemiological advice in relation to a particular animal health issue, veterinary epidemiology offers a wide range of methods which can be grouped as shown in Table 1.1. The epidemiological investigation

Table 1.1 Structured grouping of epidemiological research methods

Question	Animal health problem		
Data collection	Epidemiological studies	Surveillance and monitoring	Existing knowledge
Description	Descriptive analysis	Economic analysis	
Causal relationships	Data-driven modelling	Knowledge-driven modelling	
Intervention	Data-driven modelling	Knowledge-driven modelling	Economic analysis
Answer(s)	Control or prevention		

usually starts with the question of whether there is an animal health problem. This will require collection of data or access to and collation of existing data. The data may include a wide range of measurements including animal, management, economic and environmental factors, and they may be collected at different resolutions ranging from molecular to population level. As a first step the resulting data are analysed descriptively in terms of frequency of occurrence and possibly economic terms. These results then contribute to a decision about whether investigations of causal relationships between disease occurrence and potential risk factors are necessary to provide a science base for development of control or prevention policies. Such research into cause–effect relationships usually involves either data- or knowledge-driven modelling. The difference between these two modelling approaches is that the former is based on deriving relationships from data that have been collected, and the latter involves the development of models based on existing knowledge about the relationships within the biological system. Once the relationships are better understood, the impact of interventions can be assessed. The ultimate goal of epidemiological investigations is the control and ideally the prevention of animal disease problems by facilitating the integration of the most up-to-date scientific evidence into decision-making related to policy development.

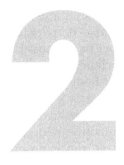

General epidemiological concepts

Learning objectives

After completing this chapter, you will be able to:

- Understand the epidemiological concepts associated with agent-host-environment and web of causation.
- Use terms utilised in infectious disease epidemiology such as infection, incubation period, reservoir, vector, pathogenicity and virulence.
- Discuss different approaches to determining cause–effect relationships.

Introduction

The basis for most epidemiological investigations is the assumption that disease does not occur in a random fashion. If it did, it would not be meaningful to investigate causal relationships between potential risk factors and disease. As discussed in Chapter 1, disease is assumed to be influenced by multiple, potentially interacting, risk factors or determinants. These can be grouped into time, place and animal characteristics. Epidemiological investigations focus on measuring these determinants for groups of animals selected from animal populations, and the defining characteristic is that both healthy and diseased animals are examined. Parameters which have to be investigated include the health status of the animal and any factors that could potentially affect its health status, such as age, body condition, vaccination status, pregnancy status, etc. The spatial and temporal location of each individual may also be relevant. Health status within a population is investigated with respect to the possible states of health of individuals, such as death, clinical or subclinical disease or health. In individual animals, disease is defined as a state of bodily function or form that fails to meet the expectations of the animal owner or society. It can manifest itself through productivity deficits or lack of quality survivorship. Genetic and molecular techniques are also now more commonly used, and they provide tools for enhanced measurement of host, agent and exposure factors.

Quantitative differences in the manifestation of infectious disease at the population level can be described using the analogy of an iceberg (see Figure 2.1). It represents the various stages with respect to infection and disease in which animals in a population will be at a particular point in time. For many infectious diseases, a substantial number of animals which were or were not exposed to infection remain uninfected and these represent the base of the iceberg. These animals may be susceptible to infection in the future, or may develop immunity as a consequence of previous exposure. Another group of animals may be infected, but has not developed clinical disease at this particular point in time. This group of animals may always remain in this category, or could at some stage develop clinical disease depending on the influence of different factors, including for example environmental stress. These animals often remain undetected by a disease surveillance system. The tip of the iceberg includes animals with different manifestations of clinical disease. The likelihood of animals in these categories being recognised through disease surveillance varies, in that those that have died or develop severe disease are usually detected, whereas those with mild illness may remain unrecognised.

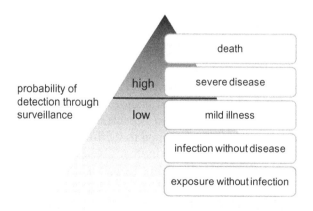

Figure 2.1   The iceberg concept of disease.

The ability of animals within these different groups to transmit infection becomes a very important factor influencing the transmission dynamics of an infectious disease, and will vary between diseases and depend on a range of risk factors.

Temporal and spatial patterns of disease

Temporal patterns of disease can be broadly categorised into epidemic and endemic disease. *Epidemics* are defined as disease occurrence which is higher than 'normal', whereas *endemicity* refers to disease which is most of the time, and therefore 'normally', present in a population. It can be difficult to distinguish between what is 'normal' disease occurrence and what not. *Pandemic* disease occurrence refers to widespread epidemics usually occurring on a global scale, such as the Spanish influenza epidemic in 1918–19. *Outbreaks* involve a sudden increase in the number of cases, and are often used to describe unusual occurrence at the herd level. *Sporadic* disease occurrence is characterised by single cases or clusters of disease which are normally not present in an area. Temporal patterns of disease are presented using bar charts showing the number of new cases on the vertical and time on the horizontal axis, and these are called epidemic curves. The shape of the epidemic curve can be used to develop hypotheses with respect to the potential cause of the disease and its epidemiological characteristics. Clustering of disease occurrence in time can be described as *short-term variation* as in the case of classical epidemics such as the UK 2001 FMD outbreak (see Figure 2.2); *periodic or seasonal variation* such as with avian influenza in Vietnam in 2004–6 (see Figure 2.3);

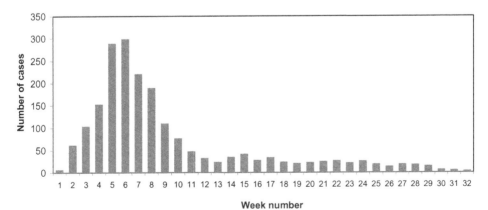

Figure 2.2   Epidemic curve for 2001 UK FMD outbreak (from Anderson 2002). With permission from The Stationery Office, UK.

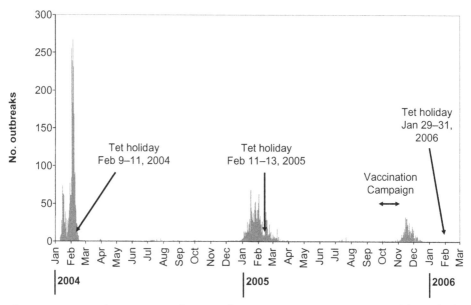

Figure 2.3 Periodic occurrence of avian influenza H5N1 in Vietnam. Reprinted from Pfeiffer *et al.* (2007). Copyright 2007, with permission from Elsevier.

and *long-term variation*, e.g. for the increasing numbers of new bovine tuberculosis herd breakdowns in the UK (Figure 2.4).

Figure 2.5 shows examples of the four standard types of curves of disease occurrence. The identification of the first case, the index case, is quite important, in that it allows inferences about infectiousness and incubation period of the disease. In the case of a *propagating epidemic*, disease is likely to have been introduced through a single source and subsequently has been transmitted from infected animals to susceptible ones within the same population. This behaviour is typical for an infectious disease with relatively short incubation period, such as foot-and-mouth disease. With *sporadic* disease occurrence only a small number of cases are observed during a short period of time, which would infer that the disease process is not infectious under the prevailing conditions. This type of pattern is usually shown by congenital deformations. In the case of a *point epidemic* a large number of new cases occur during a relatively short period of time. The key characteristic of such an epidemic is that new case numbers drop very quickly, indicating that the source of infection has been removed and no transmission between infected and susceptible animals occurs. Feed-borne causes such as toxins in animal feed may exhibit this type of behaviour. *Endemic* disease occurrence refers to the appearance of cases at all times.

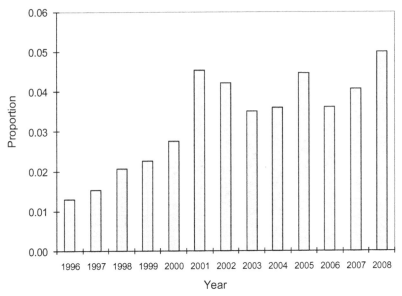

Figure 2.4 Temporal pattern of proportion of herds with positive *M. bovis* tests among previously TB-free herds (from Defra 2009). With permission from Defra.

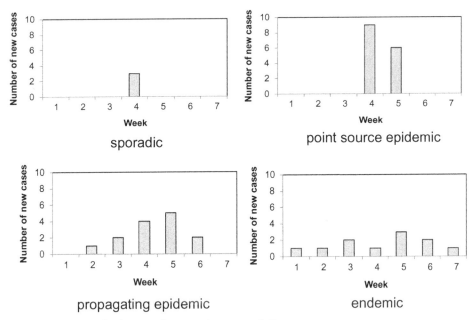

Figure 2.5 Standard types of temporal patterns of disease occurrence.

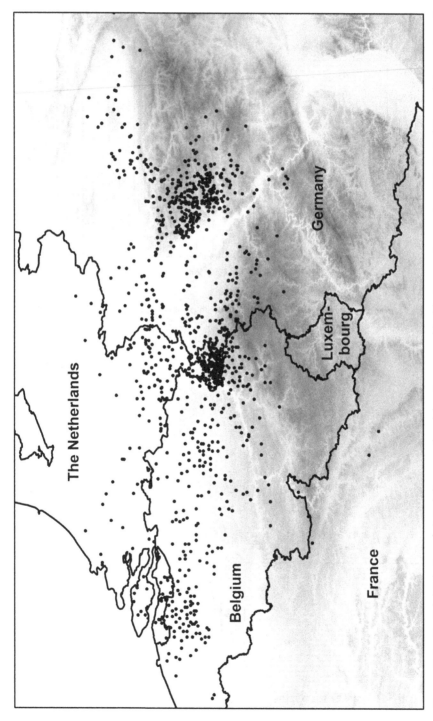

Figure 2.6 Spatial distribution of clinical disease outbreak locations caused by bluetongue virus serotype 8 in Central Europe between August and October 2006 (grey shaded background indicates height above sea level – dark higher, light lower) (from Anonymous 2006). With permission from EFSA.

Disease occurrence can also be characterised through its spatial pattern. It is usually of interest to determine whether disease occurs in a spatially clustered pattern which may be the result of transmission of infectious disease among animals in close proximity to each other or of presence of risk factors at the location of the cluster. Figure 2.6 shows the spatial distribution of disease outbreaks caused by bluetongue virus serotype 8 during August to October 2006. The virus had been introduced by an unknown mechanism into a relatively small area where Germany, the Netherlands and Belgium share borders. From here the virus was spread by *Culicoides* vector and/or animal movement predominantly in an east to west direction.

Determinants of health and disease

The concept of causation links potential risk factors with the occurrence of disease. It is further discussed in the next section of this chapter. Knowledge of these factors potentially allows control or prevention of disease. Investigations into cause–effect relationships become useful in populations where not every individual is affected by the disease under study. This involves the measurement of factors describing variation within or between husbandry systems with respect to economic, social, physical and biological parameters. They can be factors from one or more of these parameter groups, and as risk factors or determinants of health and disease, they alter the nature or frequency of disease. The term *epidemiological triad* describes the interrelationship between agent, host and environment as determinants of disease (see Figure 2.7).

Agent determinants include pathogenicity, which is the ability of an agent to produce disease in a range of hosts under a range of environmental conditions, and virulence, which is a measure of the severity of disease caused by a specific agent. The incubation period is defined as the time between infection and the first appearance of clinical signs. A major component of the epidemiology of any infectious process is the relationship between host and agent. It is characterised as being dynamic but there will often be a balance between the host's resistance mechanisms and the agent's infectivity and virulence. The agent increases its survival by increasing its infectivity and decreasing its

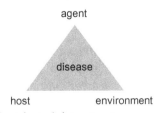

Figure 2.7 The triad of epidemiological determinants.

pathogenicity as well as through shorter generation intervals. The outcome of infection can be latent infection, clinical disease, carrier state, sterile immunity or death. A carrier state or latent infection is characterised by an infected host who is capable of disseminating the agent, but typically does not show evidence of clinical disease. Incubatory carriers, on the other hand, are infected and disseminate, but are in the preclinical stage. Convalescent carriers are infected and disseminate, but are in the postclinical stage. The agent for a particular disease can be transmitted via different mechanisms whose identification may allow introduction of specific measures for preventing transmission. These include ingestion, aerial transmission, contact, inoculation, iatrogenic and coital transmission (Thrusfield 2005). Some agents can reproduce during transmission (e.g. *Salmonella*). The presence of vectors or intermediate hosts can be a requirement for an infectious agent to survive within an ecosystem. Under such circumstances, the definitive host (usually a vertebrate) allows the agent to go through a sexual phase of development. In the intermediate host (vertebrate or invertebrate), the agent undergoes an asexual phase of development. A vector is an invertebrate actively transmitting the infectious agent between infected and susceptible vertebrates through mechanical or biological transmission. The latter can be transovarial, allowing maintenance of infection within the vector population, or trans-stadial, involving transmission between different development stages of a vector.

Host determinants include factors such as species, breed, age and sex. The range of susceptible host species varies substantially between infectious agents. Many disease agents such as *Mycobacterium bovis* can infect a larger number of different animal species. A species is considered a natural reservoir of infection if infection can be maintained within the species' population without requiring periodic reintroduction. This type of epidemiological scenario can greatly complicate control or eradication of a disease in domestic livestock, particularly if the reservoir of infection is a wildlife species. This is the case for bovine tuberculosis in several countries where infection circulates in specific wild animal reservoir species, resulting in repeated introductions of infection into domestic cattle populations (see Figure 2.8). Host susceptibility can vary between breeds of a particular animal species such as between *Bos indicus* and *Bos taurus* with respect to tick resistance. Variation in age susceptibility is probably the most important intrinsic host determinant. A key factor in this context is passive immunity which is conferred to newborn animals by their mother and may result in low incidence of infection for a disease in young animals.

Environmental determinants of disease include positional, climatic and animal husbandry factors. The geographical position, for example, is about whether a farm is in the vicinity of a wetland area with high density of wild bird species that may represent a reservoir of avian influenza infection. Climatic factors affect the distribution of vector species, e.g. *Culicoides* spp.

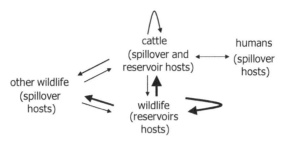

Figure 2.8 Role of different types of host species in the epidemiology of *Mycobacterium bovis* with thickness of arrows indicating relative importance of transmission between host species (from Pfeiffer (2008). Reproduced with permission of Edward Arnold (Publishers) Ltd.

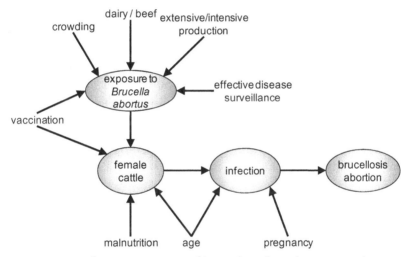

Figure 2.9 Factors influencing occurrence of bovine brucellosis abortion in cattle.

which are vectors for bluetongue virus, or whether the agent is able to survive for extended periods of time in the environment. Husbandry factors include the specific ways in which animals are being kept and fed.

Causation

The term *web of causation* is often used to describe the complex web of interacting factors involving agent, host and environment which is responsible for many diseases. Figure 2.9 shows some of the factors influencing the occurrence of bovine brucellosis abortion as an example of a web of causation (for further details see Radostits *et al.* 2007).

The *sufficient-component cause* model is useful for describing multifactorial causal mechanisms (Rothman *et al.* 2008e). *Sufficient causes* are sets of causal components that represent conditions and events which are sufficient for disease to occur. For the same disease there may be different sufficient causes. If a component appears in every sufficient cause, it is called a *necessary component cause*. For example, cattle may become infected with *Mycobacterium avium* spp. *paratuberculosis* (MAP) as calves, but most animals will never develop clinical disease involving severe wasting due to prolonged diarrhoea. In this case, the sufficient cause is still not completely understood. Infection with MAP will be a necessary causal component and other causal components are likely to be age at infection and infection dose as well as various stress factors. Figure 2.10 shows several examples of possible sufficient causes for bovine respiratory disease complex. One includes an external stressor such as cold weather, infection with viruses such as parainfluenza 3 virus (PI-3) and the bacterium *Mannheimia haemolytica* (Rice *et al.* 2007). Another involves the presence of *Pasteurella multocida* together with stress resulting from mixing of calves from several sources (Dabo *et al.* 2007), and the last links the impaired innate immune response in the lungs resulting from bovine viral diarrhoea virus (BVDV) infection with *Mycoplasma bovis* (Caswell and Archambault 2007). In general, it appears that sufficient causes for BRDC consist of component causes including one or several stressors together with specific viruses and ubiquitous bacteria. The interrelationship between the component causes as part of a sufficient cause represents an

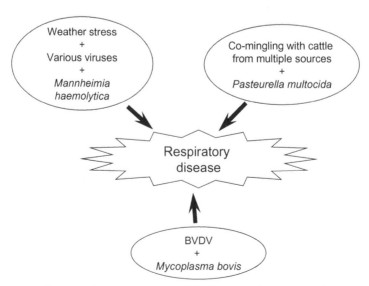

Figure 2.10 Sufficient and component causes of respiratory disease in cattle.

example of biological interaction, which has to be differentiated from statistical interaction to be discussed later.

Risk factors can be direct or indirect causes of disease. Figure 2.11 shows transport of cattle and the resulting stress as indirect causes of pneumonic pasteurellosis, whereas a direct cause will be reduced pneumonic resistance to the commensal bacterium *Mannheimia haemolytica* which is normally only present in the upper respiratory tract (Rice *et al.* 2007).

A *cause* of a disease is an event, condition, or characteristic which plays an essential role in producing an occurrence of the disease. Knowledge about such cause–effect relationships underlies every therapeutic manoeuvre in clinical medicine. Different methods are used for establishing cause, e.g. personal experience, intuition, recommendations from others or scientific evidence. The scientific principles for investigating cause–effect relationships have been a subject of research for philosophers and other scientists since ancient times. Two key doctrines from the philosophy of science are of particular relevance: induction and refutationism (Rothman 2002). *Induction* implies that generalised statements about cause and effect are derived from empirical observations made in a particular study. *Refutationism* assumes that a general statement about cause and effect can only be corroborated by every new piece of supporting evidence; it can never be proved. Instead, it can be refuted by the results from a single study indicating absence of cause and effect. When aiming to establish cause it is therefore important to realise that it is impossible to prove causal relationships beyond doubt. But it is possible to use empirical evidence to increase one's conviction of a cause–effect relationship to a point where, for all intents and purposes, cause is established and the evidence can then be used to justify therapeutic action, for example.

Different sets of criteria are used to provide evidence of cause–effect relationships. The Henle–Koch postulates developed in 1840 by Jacob Henle and expanded in 1884 by his student Robert Koch were the first set of criteria used

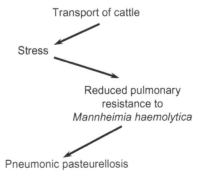

Figure 2.11   Direct and indirect causes for pneumonic pasteurellosis in cattle.

to provide a generally accepted framework for identifying causes of disease. They demanded the following rules to be met before an agent could be considered the cause of a disease:

- It has to be present in every case of the disease.
- It has to be isolated and grown in pure culture.
- It has to cause specific disease when inoculated into a susceptible animal and then be recovered from the animal and identified.

These postulates played an important role in the development of medical science until the mid 20th century. Once public health had reached a relatively high standard, it became apparent that these postulates have difficulty dealing with multiple aetiological factors, multiple effects of single causes, carrier states, non-agent factors (age, breed) and quantitative causal factors. This means that a risk factor may well be a cause of disease despite not fulfilling the Henle–Koch postulates.

Working on the basis of John Stuart Mill's rules of inductive reasoning published in 1856, both Hill (1965) and Evans (1976) independently developed sets of criteria for causation. They are very similar and have proved useful for identifying cause–effect relationships in epidemiology. Evans' criteria are presented here and they include the following:

- The proportion of individuals with the disease should be higher in those exposed to the putative cause than in those not exposed.
- The exposure to the putative cause should be more common in cases than in those without the disease.
- The number of new cases should be higher in those exposed to the putative cause than in those not exposed, as shown in prospective studies.
- Temporally, the disease should follow exposure to the putative cause.
- There should be a measurable biological spectrum of host responses.
- The host response should be repeatable following exposure to the putative cause.
- The disease should be reproducible experimentally more frequently in those animals which are exposed to the putative cause than in those not.
- Preventing or modifying the host response should decrease or eliminate the expression of disease.
- Elimination of the putative cause should result in a lower incidence of the disease.
- The relationship should be biologically and epidemiologically plausible.

If a risk factor or determinant fails to fulfil one or more of the above criteria (except for the fourth – temporality), this does not exclude the possibility that a causal relationship exists. And if a factor fulfils all criteria, it is still possible that it may not be a cause.

Although the concepts presented above are now fairly well established, it is important to be aware of the impact of molecular and genetic methods for host and pathogen characterisation on approaches for establishment of cause–effect relationships. In this context, the following short list of publications can be used to obtain further information:

- Falkow (2004) proposed a set of molecular Koch's postulates.
- Fredericks and Relman (1996) adapted Evans' postulates for use with nucleic acid sequence data.
- Lipkin (2008) refers to the opportunities and challenge represented by the increasing rate of the discovery of new pathogens.
- Both Page *et al.* (2003) and Khoury *et al.* (2008) discuss causation in association with gene–disease association studies.

Quantifying disease occurrence

Learning objectives

After completing this chapter, you will be able to:

- Correctly calculate and interpret risk and rate measures of disease frequency.
- Understand the meaning of survival probability and hazard rate.
- Standardise disease risks and rates by taking account of confounding factors.

Introduction

One of the most fundamental tasks in epidemiological research is the quantification of disease occurrence. The event of interest may be infection, clinical disease or death at the individual animal level, but it is also possible to use the disease status of aggregates of animals, such as herds. It is important to provide a clear case definition and description of the population within which the cases occurred, since otherwise the data may not be appropriately interpreted by others.

Counts, ratios, proportions and rates are the main mathematical quantities used for describing disease occurrence. *Counts* are an enumeration of the number of cases. *Ratios* are mathematical expressions relating one quantity to another. A *proportion* is a ratio in which the numerator is included within the denominator. It has no units, ranges from 0 to 1 and is often expressed as a percentage after multiplication by 100. *Rates* are ratios which express change in one type of quantity relative to change in another kind of quantity.

Rates have units and do not have a finite upper bound. An example is the heart rate or the speed of a car.

A count of the number of animals which are infected, diseased, or dead may be useful for estimating workload, cost, or size of facilities to provide health care, but is of limited value for epidemiological research. It is often easier to obtain counts of diseased than of healthy animals, particularly when the population that is to be followed up over time is open, meaning animals can be added or removed during that time, rather than closed. A count can also be expressed as a proportion of the number of animals capable of experiencing infection, disease or death. The latter is also called the *population* or, if a group of non-diseased animals is followed up over time (= follow-up period), the *population at risk*. The concept of *risk* is also important. This defines the probability that disease develops in an individual animal during a specific period of time, and is calculated as a proportion.

Disease frequency based only on new (= incident) cases of disease can be quantified using incidence (incidence risk and rate) or survival measures (survival and hazard function), thereby describing disease onset. The animals to be included must be healthy at the beginning of the observation period. Each animal is then followed over time until it develops the disease or until its observation period finishes (e.g. sold or end of study period). The reference event defining the starting point of the observation period can be an event specific to each animal, such as birth, treatment or date of introduction to the herd, or it can be a common calendar date for the population under study, e.g. the start date of a study. The associated calculations may also include the same animal developing disease repeatedly as long as recovery within the follow-up period can be assumed. Old as well as new (= prevalent) cases are included in the calculation of the prevalence which means that health status rather than its change is measured. The statistical uncertainty associated with these measures of disease occurrence can be expressed by calculating confidence intervals for the point estimates of risks and rates. Chapter 6 presents the relevant mathematical calculations for proportions. Morris and Gardner (2000) focus on confidence interval calculations for different types of epidemiological outcome parameters.

Incidence risk

The risk of new disease occurrence is quantified using *incidence risk*, also called cumulative incidence, incidence proportion, case fatality rate or attack rate. It is defined as the proportion of disease-free individuals developing a given disease over a specified time. Note that animals have to be disease-free at the beginning of the follow-up period to be included in the numerator or denominator of this calculation. Incidence risk is interpreted as an individual's risk of contracting or developing disease within the follow-up period. For diseases where animals can develop the same disease several times during the follow-up period, only the first event can be counted. The quantity has no units, ranges from 0 to 1 and is not interpretable without specification of the time period. It assumes a closed population, i.e. no animal leaves or enters the population during the period of follow-up. If a small number of animals are removed during the study, the population at risk can be adjusted by subtracting half the number of withdrawn animals (this assumes that on average animals are removed in the middle of the study period). A limitation of incidence risk, particularly with long study periods and a specific cause of death as an outcome, is that animals will be exposed to multiple or competing risks, and it will therefore be difficult to obtain accurate risk estimates. As an example for an incidence risk calculation, a herd of 121 cattle is tested using the tuberculin test and all test negative. One year later, the same 121 cattle are tested again (i.e. no animals have been removed or added) and 25 test positive. The incidence risk over a period of 12 months can then be calculated as 25/121, which amounts to 0.21 (= 21%). Hence, a randomly selected animal from this herd had a 21% chance of becoming infected over the 12 month period.

Incidence rate

Incidence rate quantifies the number of cases to be expected per unit of animal time. The terms incidence density, hazard rate, force of morbidity or mortality are also used. The incidence rate is not a risk or probability, and therefore does not have an interpretation at the individual animal level. Instead it is an instantaneous concept, meaning that the calculated value expresses the rate at which cases are occurring at a given instant. In that sense it is similar to the speed of a car which can be expressed in km/hour, but still relates to the speed at a particular moment (Rothman 2002). Incidence rate is calculated using the number of new cases observed over the follow-up period in the numerator and the accumulated sum of all individuals' time at risk in the denominator. The time at risk contributed by each animal is the time from start of follow-up until disease occurs, until the animal is removed from the population or the follow-up period has finished. In contrast to incidence risk, incidence rate allows us to deal with competing risks, in that an animal which dies from a different cause or develops a disease other than the one studied can still contribute the time period during which it was at risk of developing the disease of interest. Individual animals can contribute several time periods to numerator and denominator, from the time when they recovered from the previous disease occurrence. Incidence rate has units of inverse time, a lower bound of zero and no upper bound. An exact or an approximate denominator can be used for its calculation. The exact denominator is based on the sum of animal time units during which each animal was at risk. The approximate denominator uses the total number of disease-free animals (or its product with the follow-up period) at the start of the follow-up period, from which ½ of diseased animals, ½ of withdrawn animals and ½ of added animals are subtracted (Dohoo *et al.* 2009). The numeric quantity produced by the incidence rate calculation is meaningful only in the context of the time units it relates to. The time units can be adjusted by multiplication of the numeric quantity, and having at least one digit to the left of the decimal place is recommended. Incidence rates have several limitations. One is that they only allow calculation of average rates over a time period, and therefore may hide temporal patterns. Also, the total animal time at risk does not differentiate between animals that only contributed short periods at risk and those which may have been followed up for a long time. Another limitation is that the same numeric quantity could be obtained from very different size study groups or samples, thereby complicating interpretation. For example, an incidence rate of 1 diseased case per 100 animal weeks can be obtained from following 100 animals on average for 1 week or from 2 animals for 100 weeks together.

As an example for an incidence rate calculation, a study was conducted over a period of 12 months to determine the mortality of cows in a village which has a total of 100 cows at the beginning of the study.

- 5 cows die after 2 months, which means together they were $5 \times 2 = 10$ animal months at risk.
- 2 cows die after 5 months, which means together they were $2 \times 5 = 10$ animal months at risk.
- 3 cows die after 8 months, which means together they were $3 \times 8 = 24$ animal months at risk.

This means a total of 10 cows die, and these experienced 44 animal months at risk based on the above calculation.

- 90 cows survive past the study period which means they were 90×12 months = 1080 animal months at risk.

Therefore, the incidence rate for cow mortality in this village using the exact denominator method is calculated as $10/1124 = 0.009$ deaths per animal month, or 9 deaths per 1000 animal months at risk.

Prevalence

The proportion of a population affected by a disease at a given point in time is called *prevalence*. It is also referred to as prevalence rate or prevalence proportion. *Point prevalence* describes disease occurrence at a single point in time and *period prevalence* over a period of time. Prevalence can be interpreted as the probability of a randomly selected individual from this or a similar population having the disease at this point in time. It is therefore very important for diagnostic decision-making. The prevalent disease cases used in the numerator include old as well as new cases. This means that diseases with low incidence rates but long survival may actually result in relatively high prevalence values, and vice versa. Prevalence is of limited use for aetiological research of diseases associated with long duration, as it cannot differentiate between factors that affect disease occurrence and survival of diseased animals.

As an example of a prevalence calculation, assume a situation where blood samples are taken from a herd of 173 dairy cows to assess the frequency of *Neospora caninum* infection. If 15 of these animals test positive, the prevalence can be calculated as 15/173 amounting to 0.09 (9%). This means that a randomly selected dairy cow from this herd has a 9% chance of being infected at this point in time.

Comparison of prevalence and incidence measures

When comparing incidence risk and prevalence, it is important to realise that only the first includes a temporal sequence. Incidence risk includes only new cases in the numerator, whereas prevalence does not distinguish between old and new cases. Incidence risk predicts what will be happening in the future, i.e. the probability that similar individuals will develop the condition. This is useful for making decisions about preventive measures such as vaccination. Prevalence describes the probability of having the disease among a group of animals, usually at a point in time. Every clinician uses this information during the clinical decision-making process. Both measures can be used to make comparisons between risk factors, but incidence risk is more appropriate, as it is not affected by disease duration. Table 3.1 presents a comparison of the three methods expressing disease frequency.

Figure 3.1 shows a comparative example of prevalence and incidence calculations. It is based on a population of 10 animals which are followed up over a 12 month period with each of them being healthy at the start. For animals that are diagnosed with disease or withdrawn in a given month, the time at risk is assumed to finish with the previous month. For example, animal A shows disease in May and therefore was at risk from January until April; animal C was withdrawn from the population in August which means that it was at risk of becoming diseased from January to July. In total, 4 animals develop disease and 2 are withdrawn from the study. The prevalence proportions express the probability of an animal being diseased in the respective month, 0.33 and 0.5 respectively. It is an example of a seasonal pattern of

Table 3.1   Comparison of incidence and prevalence measures

	Incidence rate	Incidence risk	Prevalence
Numerator	New cases occurring during a period of time among a group initially free of disease	New cases occurring during a period of time among a group initially free of disease	All cases counted during a single survey of a group
Denominator	Sum of time periods during which individuals could have developed disease	All susceptible individuals present at the beginning of the period	All individuals examined, including cases and non-cases
Time	For each individual from beginning of follow-up until disease	Duration of the period	Single point or period
Interpretation	Number of new cases per unit of time	Risk of developing disease over a given time period	Probability of having disease at a particular point in time

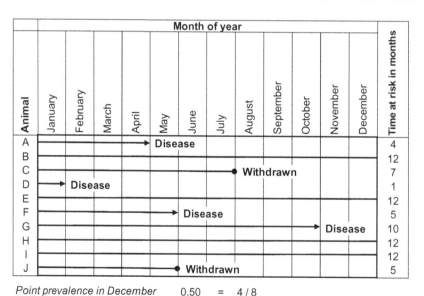

Point prevalence in December	0.50	=	4 / 8
Point prevalence in June	0.33	=	3 / 9
Incidence risk per year			
exact denominator	0.50	=	4 / 8
approximate denominator	0.44	=	4 /(10 - 0.5 * 2)
Incidence rate per animal year			
exact denominator	0.60	=	4 / ((4 + 12 + 7 + 1 + 12 + 5 + 10 + 12 + 12 + 5)/12)
approximate denominator	0.57	=	4 /(10 - 0.5 * 4 - 0.5 * 2)

Figure 3.1   Example calculation for prevalence and incidence measures of disease occurrence.

prevalence, since the calculated numeric values as well as the denominators are different for June and December. Incidence risk has been calculated both using an exact denominator where only the animals are included which were available for follow-up for the complete study period, and using an approximate denominator where half the withdrawals are subtracted. The resulting values of 0.5 and 0.44 express the risk of an animal developing disease per 12 months or 1 year, since that was the length of the follow-up period. Incidence rate has also been calculated with two denominators, and in units of animal years, rather than months for ease of comparison with the prevalence and incidence risk values calculated (note that this is the reason why the exact denominator value has been divided by 12 months). It is important to remember that these incidence rate values do not express a risk or probability, but rather the number of cases to be expected per year, in this example 0.6 or 0.57 cases per year.

Miscellaneous measures of disease occurrence

Other measures of disease frequency, some of which have already been mentioned above, include the *attack rate* which is defined as the number of new cases divided by the initial population at risk. It is actually an incidence risk, and despite its name it is in fact a probability and not a rate. The attack rate is used when the period at risk is short.

Mortality rates are applied using a number of different interpretations, and often do not represent true rates. The *crude mortality rate* has death as the outcome of interest and is calculated analogous to incidence rate. The *cause-specific mortality* rate is estimated for specific causes of death and also calculated analogous to incidence rate. *Case fatality rate* represents the proportion of animals with a specific disease that die from it. It is a risk measure, not a rate, and is used to describe the impact of epidemics or the severity of acute disease.

Survival or time-to-event

A key parameter of interest in epidemiological research is the time until the occurrence of events such as death, infection, onset of clinical disease or recovery from it. The term *survival* is often used for this type of data, mainly because the methods were first developed for investigating mortality. It can be estimated if repeated measurements on the same group of animals are available. One characteristic of such data is usually that some animals will not develop the event of interest during the follow-up period, a process called *right censoring*. Figure 3.2 shows an example of such data. There are several options for quantifying time-to-event for a group of animals. If one were to use the

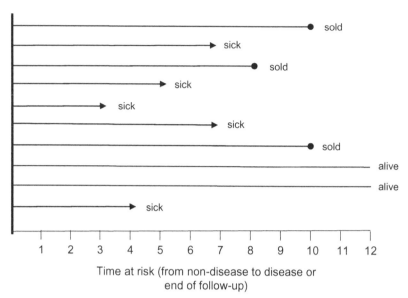

Figure 3.2 Example of time-to-event data (event = becoming sick).

average of the time-to-event, the animals which did not experience the event of interest could not be included. In Figure 3.2, they would be the ones that were sold or alive at the end of the study period. This method therefore has the disadvantage that the estimate will depend on the length of the time period over which data were collected. If the interval is too short, survival time is likely to be underestimated, and if it is very long a small number of animals with long time-to-event may have a strong influence on the mean estimate. Another option is to calculate the median time-to-event, but this can only be computed if at least 50% of animals experience the event during the follow-up period. It is also possible to calculate the incidence rate, but this calculation assumes that the rate at which the event occurs is constant throughout the period of study which very often is not the case.

The most appropriate measures for summarising the disease occurrence information in these types of data are the survivor and hazard functions. As noted above, these apply to any time-to-event data, but were first developed for investigating survival. The *survivor function* (= cumulative survival probability) is a representation of the distributional pattern of the cumulative proportion of individuals not having experienced the event (e.g. disease, death or recovery) over a given time at risk. The survivor function is non-increasing, starts with a value of 1, and can reach a minimum of 0. It is often summarised using the median survival time which is the time at which 50% of individuals at risk have experienced the event of interest. The *hazard function* is a representation of the distributional pattern of the hazard rate (= instantaneous

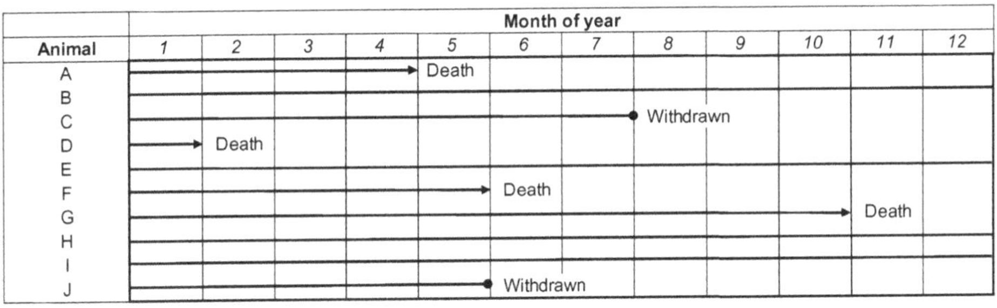

	1	2	3	4	5	6	7	8	9	10	11	12
Removed	0	0	0	0	0	1	0	1	0	0	0	0
Events	0	1	0	0	1	1	0	0	0	0	1	0
At risk	10	10	9	9	9	8	6	6	5	5	5	4
Duration	1	1	1	1	1	1	1	1	1	1	1	1
Conditional survival probability	1.00	0.90	1.00	1.00	0.89	0.88	1.00	1.00	1.00	1.00	0.80	1.00
Conditional event probability	0.00	0.10	0.00	0.00	0.11	0.13	0.00	0.00	0.00	0.00	0.20	0.00
Hazard rate	0.00	0.10	0.00	0.00	0.11	0.13	0.00	0.00	0.00	0.00	0.20	0.00
Cumulative survival probability	1.00	0.90	0.90	0.90	0.80	0.70	0.70	0.70	0.70	0.70	0.56	0.56

Figure 3.3 Example calculation for survivor and hazard functions.

failure rate, force of mortality, conditional mortality rate, age-specific failure rate). The latter is calculated by dividing the probability of an animal experiencing the event of interest during a specific time interval, given it has not experienced it prior to that time, by the length of the specified time interval. The key advantages of the survivor and hazard function are as follows. The calculations can make use of right-censored observations, i.e. animals that did not experience the event of interest during the follow-up period. The resulting quantities are risks and rates which have a convenient interpretation in epidemiological research. It is also possible to use non-parametric approaches for the calculations, so that no assumptions about the shape of the distributions are necessary.

An example calculation for survival data is presented in Figure 3.3. Animal A survived for 4 months, B survived the whole period of 12 months, C was removed from the population after 7 months, and so on. For the calculations, it is assumed that the event of interest in these data (i.e. death) has occurred some time during the last month under observation (i.e. in month 4 for animal A), and that withdrawn animals were at risk until the end of the last month of observation (i.e. animal C was at risk until month 7 inclusive). The row labelled 'At risk' shows the number of animals at risk during a particular month, i.e. animals that have died in the previous month or were withdrawn at the end of the previous month have been subtracted. The rows for 'Events'

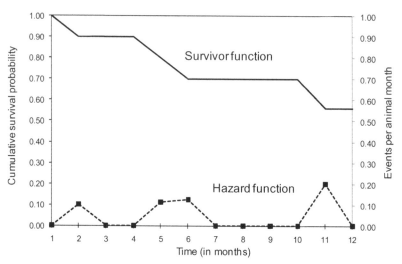

Figure 3.4 Plots for survivor and hazard functions based on the example calculation (survivor function relates to y-axis on the left, hazard function to y-axis on the right).

and 'Removed' represent the animals that were withdrawn or died, respectively. The 'Events' row is used as the numerator and the 'At risk' row as the denominator for the calculation of the conditional survival probability during a particular month. The product of the conditional survival probabilities expresses the cumulative survival probability. The hazard rate is the quotient between the row 'Conditional event probability' in a particular time interval (i.e. 1 – conditional survival probability) and the row 'Duration' representing the length of the respective follow-up interval (i.e. 1 month in this case). The resulting graphs for the survivor and hazard functions based on the values for cumulative survival probability and hazard rate, respectively, are shown in Figure 3.4.

Standardisation of occurrence measures

An overall risk or rate estimate for a population as an aggregated quantity is influenced by differences in risk or rate between population subgroups (= risk factor strata) and the relative contribution of each of these subgroups (= strata) to the total study group. Therefore, if one finds differences in overall risk or rate estimates when comparing different populations or study groups, it is unclear whether this is the result of differences in the distribution of its members across the risk factor subgroups within each population or a true difference in risk or rate between the two populations. The risk factor defining the strata within the population or study group is called a *potential confound-*

ing factor. If the potential confounder is known and of a categorical nature, an adjustment of each of the crude risks or rates can be made by introducing a differential weighting for each stratum, a process called *standardisation*. The two main methods available for performing these adjustments are direct and indirect standardisation. Note that these methods are only relevant if there are differences between the stratum-specific risk or rate estimates in a particular population or study group. Both methods use values from a standard or reference population which may be, for example, based on census data. The somewhat arbitrary choice of reference distribution will influence the standardised overall risk or rate estimate, and some epidemiologists therefore prefer to avoid this process and report only stratum-specific risk estimates (Rothman 2002). But if comparisons of risk or rate estimates have to be made between populations or study groups, it may be necessary to use standardisation or other analytical approaches such as Mantel–Haenszel tests or logistic regression to control for the confounding factor.

Direct standardisation

Direct standardisation involves weighting a set of observed stratum-specific risk or rate estimates according to a predefined standard distribution. This approach should only be used when large sample sizes are available. First, stratum-specific risks or rates are calculated. The direct standardised risk or rate estimate is then obtained as the sum of the products across the strata between the proportion of the standard population in stratum *i* and the observed risk or rate estimate in stratum *i* in the overall population or study group. As an example (see Figure 3.5), assuming that mortality in cats is influenced by the risk factors obesity and being kept indoors, any comparison of mortality between cats that are obese and those that are not may be influenced by the relative distribution of cats kept indoors among the two groups. In this hypothetical example, it is also assumed that obesity and being kept indoors are not associated. In fact, it appears that the crude mortality risk is lower for obese cats (0.14 per year) than it is for cats that are not obese (0.22 per year). In this example, the stratum-specific mortality risks were re-weighted using 0.2 for the cats kept indoors and 0.8 for those that were not, and the

	Indoors	Animals	Deaths	Stratum-specific mortality risk per year	Crude mortality risk per year	Weighting	Direct standardised mortality risk per year
Obese	yes	40	4	0.10	0.14	0.20	0.26
	no	10	3	0.30		0.80	
Not obese	yes	20	1	0.05	0.22	0.20	0.21
	no	100	25	0.25		0.80	

Figure 3.5 Example of direct standardisation calculations.

resulting direct standardised mortality risks are now more similar between obese and non-obese cats. In this example, the previously observed difference was the result of the difference in the relative distribution of indoor cats among obese and non-obese cats, i.e. a much higher proportion of obese than of non-obese cats was kept indoors.

Indirect standardisation

In order to be able to use indirect standardisation, we need to have stratum-specific risk or rate estimates for the standard population and the distribution of the adjusting factor in the study group. The method can be used either if stratum-specific risk or rate estimates are not available for the study group, as long as the overall risk can be calculated, or if the stratum-specific estimates are available but are based on small sample sizes. As a first step, an expected number of cases is calculated on the basis of the sum of the products between standard stratum-specific risks or rates and observed stratum-specific numbers of animals or animal-time in the study group. The *standardised morbidity* or *mortality ratio* (SMR) is based on dividing the observed by the expected number of cases. The indirect standardised risk or rate can be obtained through multiplication of the SMR with the overall risk or rate from the standard population.

The example in Figure 3.6 uses the same data as for the direct standardisation above. The standard population assumes a mortality risk of 0.05 per year for cats kept indoors and 0.2 per year otherwise, and the overall mortality risk in the standard population is assumed to be 0.17 per year. The observed mortality among obese cats is 7 deaths. The expected number of cases among obese cats ($n = 4$) was obtained by summing the products between the number of animals kept indoors ($n = 40$) and the respective standard stratum-specific mortality risk of 0.05 on the one hand and the proportion kept outdoors ($n = 10$) and the corresponding stratum-specific mortality risk of 0.2 on the other. The standardised mortality ratio for obese cats is calculated as the ratio

	Indoors	Animals	Observed deaths per year	Crude mortality risk per year	Standard stratum-specific & overall mortality risk per year	Expected deaths per year	SMR	Indirect standardised mortality risk per year
Obese	yes	40			0.05			
	no	10			0.20			
	total	50	7	0.14	0.17	4	1.75	0.30
Not obese	yes	20			0.05			
	no	100			0.20			
	total	120	26	0.22	0.17	21	1.24	0.21

Figure 3.6 Example calculation for indirect standardisation.

between observed (n = 7) and expected mortality (n = 4), resulting in an SMR of 1.75. An indirect standardised mortality risk of 0.3 per year was calculated as the product between the overall mortality risk in the standard population (0.17) and the SMR (1.75). The resulting figure is very different for obese cats, as a result of the proportion of cats kept indoors being different from that of the standard population.

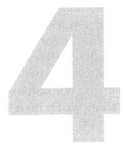

Designing epidemiological studies

Learning objectives

After completing this chapter, you will be able to:

- Design an experimental or observational epidemiological study.
- Understand the differences between as well as advantages/disadvantages of the different study designs.

Introduction

As discussed in Chapter 1, the major aims of epidemiology are to describe the health status of populations, to explain the aetiology of diseases, to predict disease occurrence and to control the distribution of disease. Any of these aims will require access to data for analysis. The data may already have been collected, e.g. as part of a disease surveillance programme, or need to be collected through a specifically designed study. If the data have not yet been collected, it needs to be clear what the target and source population are. The *target population* is the population to which the results from the study are to be generalised. The *source population* is the one from which the actual units of study, such as animals or herds, have been selected. The *study group* or *sample* consists of the individual study units that have been selected. A more detailed discussion of these concepts is presented in Chapter 7.

Epidemiological studies can be categorised into descriptive and analytical studies. Case reports, case series and surveys are examples of *descriptive studies. Analytical* or *explanatory studies* include experimental and observational studies. They involve comparison between groups of animals with respect to the statistical association between one or several risk factors and an outcome of interest, such as disease status, and thereby allow inferences with respect to cause–effect relationships. With any of the different types of analytical studies it needs to be kept in mind that all phenomena within biological systems are interrelated, which complicates the situation for an investigator who will have to select a segment of the whole system for the study or attempt to represent it in a laboratory. The various types of analytical studies differ with respect to the balance achieved between optimal control of measurement and representing the 'real world'. The *experimental study* is at one end of the spectrum, considering that it allows good control of measurement and study conditions, but it may be less likely to represent the 'real world'. The *observational study* is at the opposite end, allowing less control over the study conditions and measurement, but being more likely to represent the 'real world'. *Ecological observational studies* are based on study units which are an aggregate of the unit of interest. The aggregates could be herds or farms, for example, despite the aim of the research being to identify risk factors for individual animals. Any inferences from such studies need to be interpreted very cautiously, because the results are potentially subject to a bias known as the *ecological fallacy*. The key issue here is that risk factors operating at the aggregate level may not have affected every individual within the study units.

Systematic reviews and *meta-analyses* could be considered to belong to the group of analytical studies. They differ from narrative literature reviews, in that they involve a structured synthesis of published scientific evidence – quantitative in the case of meta-analysis. These are considered to provide the best evidence for cause–effect relationships, and are therefore of particular relevance in evidence-based veterinary medicine (Cockcroft and Holmes 2003).

Descriptive studies

Both case reports and case series focus on individual sick animals and have long been at the centre of clinical knowledge. They are based on direct personal observation relating to anatomical structure and physiological function, which can be quantified and be systematic but usually is largely qualitative. Although these observations can be extremely intensive and detailed, their main disadvantage for assessing cause–effect relationships is that they do not involve comparison. Surveys are also descriptive and often involve random selection of a sample from a source population. They aim to describe disease frequency, but do not collect data on risk factors.

Experimental studies

An experimental study involves manipulation of the conditions of study (i.e. application of an intervention), and can be conducted either in a controlled environment, such as a laboratory, or in the natural environment of the animals (= field). If it is conducted as an experimental laboratory study, great precision in measurement and optimal control of influencing variables can be achieved, resulting in sound cause–effect inferences. The disadvantage is that in a laboratory it is usually not possible to represent the myriad of factors affecting disease occurrence in an animal's natural environment, and it may be difficult to work with sufficient numbers of animals to represent true variation between animals in the natural population. If an experimental study is conducted in the natural environment of the animals, it is called an *experimental field study* (= controlled trial, clinical trial or intervention study). In contrast to the laboratory experiment, the animals will be exposed to all known and unknown factors present in their natural environment. These studies are usually used to evaluate therapeutic or preventive effects of particular interventions, but are also useful for investigating aetiological relationships.

Experimental studies typically involve dividing a group of animals into at least two subgroups: one to which an intervention will be applied and another so-called control or comparison group that will not receive the intervention (see Figure 4.1). The decision to apply an intervention to a particular animal within the study or not should be based on random allocation (= randomisation). Such a study is also called a *randomised controlled trial* (RCT). After a period of time, the status with respect to the outcome variable (e.g. disease status) is assessed for each animal. Summary measures of the response (e.g. incidence risk) are then compared between both subgroups. Differences in the summary values indicate an association between the intervention and outcome, and may therefore be suggestive of the presence of an effect of the intervention on the outcome variable.

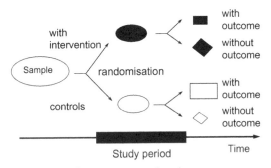

Figure 4.1   Schematic structure of an experimental study.

The effect of drugs is usually evaluated in three phases of trials (Fletcher and Fletcher 2005).

- Phase I trials focus on establishing safe dose range and identifying severe side effects, and may involve only a small number of animals without a control.
- Phase II trials address drug efficacy and the relationship between dose and efficacy. They may be controlled, but will still involve relatively small numbers of animals, and therefore detect only large effects.
- Phase III trials provide the definitive information in relation to effect and common side effects, and have to be conducted as RCTs with sufficient numbers of animals so that clinically important treatment effects can be detected.

Uncontrolled experiments describe disease behaviour in the same group of animals before and after intervention. They assume that any changes in disease subsequent to treatment are due to the treatment, which is very rarely the case. The investigators need to be aware of effects such as regression to the mean and predictable improvement. Many biological parameters, e.g. blood biochemistry, are subject to significant natural variation even in the healthy animal, and therefore a non-diseased animal may present values outside the 'normal' range at one sampling occasion, although infrequently. On subsequent measurements, the values are usually back within the 'normal' range, an effect called regression to the mean. The danger with this type of effect is that the 'improvement' may be attributed to the intervention, when in reality the treated animal had never been truly 'abnormal'. Furthermore, most diseases will improve over time, e.g. due to the immune response of the affected animal, so that improvement is predictable, and therefore the intervention may not have caused the improvement in an uncontrolled experiment.

An *experimental field study* provides the researcher with effective control over the study situation, thereby limiting the influence of various potential sources of bias. Randomisation should ensure that all factors associated with the outcome other than the intervention are equally distributed between the study subgroups. This should definitely be the case if the sample size is large enough, even if these factors are not measurable or known. If large sample sizes are not possible, control of such factors can be achieved by defining homogeneous subgroups or strata with respect to the status of these variables (= blocking or matching) within which treatment is then allocated randomly. Another option is to conduct a *cross-over study* where each animal will be in the intervention group at one time during the study and in the control group at another time. This approach can be used provided that the intervention has only a very short-lasting effect which has disappeared by the time an animal changes to the other study subgroup. Blinding or masking means that the owners of the study animals will not know which subgroup (intervention or control) the study animals are in. This will minimise the possibility of owners changing the management or handling of the animals depending on whether they are in one group or another. Experimental field studies are considered the method of choice for investigation of causal hypotheses about the effectiveness of preventive measures. Compared with observational studies they provide much better control over confounders and therefore can give stronger evidence about causality. If an experimental field study is appropriately designed, there is less opportunity for bias due to selection or misinformation compared with observational studies. They are also among one of the study designs most suitable for inclusion in systematic reviews. The disadvantages of experimental field studies are that they often require large groups, they can be costly, the required duration can be long if disease incidence is low, and selection bias may be introduced if they are not designed appropriately. A detailed description of experimental studies is provided in Dohoo *et al.* (2009).

Observational studies

An observational study is conducted in the natural environment of the animals, and involves only measurement or observation of naturally occurring events. It is one of the most frequently used techniques in epidemiological research. These studies can be conducted using prospective or retrospective data collection. With a *prospective* observational study, the data will be collected after the study has been designed, but existing data sources may also be included. In case of a *retrospective* design, information about either the outcome or the risk factors should already be available. The most important observational study designs are the cohort, the case–control and the cross-sectional studies.

Cohort study

The cohort study (= longitudinal study) is based on selecting at least two subgroups of non-diseased animals with different exposure status in relation to risk factors postulated to cause a disease (see Figure 4.2). It is also possible to select a sample or study group of animals likely to be heterogeneous with respect to risk factor levels and then determine their exposure status. In a prospective cohort study, the selected sample of animals (= cohort) is then followed over time and any animal's change in disease status is recorded during the study period. On completion of the study, incidence measures can then be compared between exposure status groups. The unit of interest in the study can be an individual animal, but it is also possible to involve groups or aggregates such as animal litters or herds. The only difference with a retrospective cohort study is that all data will be collected from past records.

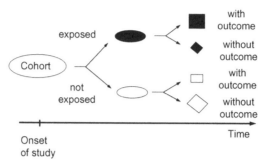

Figure 4.2 Schematic diagram of a prospective cohort study.

Exactly as with experimental studies, when assessing the relationship between a risk factor and disease in a cohort study, it is important that the different exposure groups for a particular risk factor are similar with respect to any other factors associated with that risk factor and the outcome (= confounding factors). This is unlikely to be the case without specific measures being taken during study design or analysis that will control for any such differences (Fletcher and Fletcher 2005). Randomisation would be the best approach, but it cannot be applied in an observational study. *Restricted sampling* would involve only focusing the study on a group of animals which have the same or a similar status in relation to important confounding factors. The disadvantage of this approach is that the findings from the study might be less generalisable. An alternative is *matching*, where exposed and non-exposed animals are grouped according to confounding factor status, either on a one-on-one or one-on-many basis (e.g. same age or breed) or as larger groups. This approach will only control for bias caused by the factors used to match, and for practical reasons these can usually only be relatively few. Another disadvantage of matching is that the effect of the matching factor can no longer be analysed. Alternatively, confounding factors which have been measured can be controlled for in the analysis, using standardisation, stratification or multivariable adjustment. Standardisation has been discussed in Chapter 3 under standardisation of disease occurrence measures. *Stratification* involves presenting and analysing the data as subgroups with similar characteristics, often in a tabular format. Although the results are easy to understand, this method may result in small numbers of observations in some of the strata. *Multivariable adjustment* using regression methods is less transparent, but more efficient than standardisation or stratification as it allows control for multiple confounding variables simultaneously and can handle small numbers of observations in subgroups.

A well-designed cohort study has a number of advantages. It is the most effective of the observational studies for investigation of causal hypotheses with respect to disease occurrence. It provides disease incidence estimates which are more meaningful than prevalence data for assessing cause–effect relationships, and multiple outcomes can be studied simultaneously. Cohort studies can be used to study rare exposures, and through appropriate design it is possible to minimise selection and confounding bias. Disadvantages of cohort studies include long study duration or large groups are necessary in the case of rare disease. In the case of long study duration, the potential for confounding effects increases and the ability to demonstrate causality may be compromised. Losses to follow-up or animals changing between exposure categories can become an important problem, particularly with studies of long duration. Cohort studies are also often quite expensive.

Case–control study

In a case–control study, animals with the disease (= cases) and without (= controls) are selected (see Figure 4.3). The frequency of exposure to potential risk factors is measured retrospectively for the two groups. The relative frequency of the exposure is then compared between the two groups. It is preferable to select new (or incident) rather than prevalent cases of the disease. Risk factors for prevalent disease may be associated with disease risk or duration, or both, and these effects could then not be distinguished from each other in a case–control study. All cases may be included, or a representative sample. A key requirement for case–control studies is that controls and cases need to have had a similar opportunity of exposure. This can be difficult to achieve if cases have been selected from subpopulations such as referral practices or hospitals. Ideally, controls are a random sample of non-cases from the same source population from which the cases were obtained. These are called *population-based* or *primary-base* case–control studies. If controls have to be selected from subpopulations such as referral practices or hospitals, special care needs to be taken to ensure comparability with cases. Here, a *secondary source population* or *secondary base* needs to be defined, which should

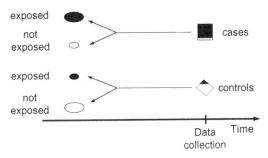

Figure 4.3 Schematic diagram of a case–control study.

represent the population that has generated the cases. If it is difficult to obtain comparable controls from a suitable source population, it is also possible to select multiple control groups, each representing different populations. If a disease is rare, and there are therefore only few cases, the ability of the study to detect important risk factors (= statistical power) can be increased by using multiple controls for each case. The selection of the controls from the primary or secondary base depends on whether a risk- or a rate-based case–control study design is used. In a *risk-based design*, controls are selected from the animals that did not develop the disease until the end of the risk period. This requires a closed population, i.e. one with no significant losses or additions. This approach is most suitable for outbreak investigations, where the risk period is short, has ended and almost all cases have occurred. Selection among the controls should involve equal sampling fractions in exposed and non-exposed animals. If the study group is open, i.e. animals are added and removed during the risk period, and/or the risk period is long, a *rate-based design* should be used for control selection, meaning that the time at risk will be taken into account. Here, the sampling rate among exposed and non-exposed controls, i.e. the ratios of exposed controls per exposed animal-time and non-exposed per non-exposed animal-time, should be similar.

As with other study designs, the validity of case–control studies depends on the extent to which confounding factors have been controlled. The approaches of restricted sampling, matching and multivariable adjustment discussed above under cohort studies can be applied. Matching needs to be used very cautiously, since any association between risk factors of interest and confounders may result in bias through overmatching (Dohoo *et al.* 2009).

The term *nested case–control study* is used when the study is conducted within a well-defined cohort where all cases are known and the non-cases are enumerated. If large databases with complete population records are available, a *case–cohort study* could be conducted which combines the ability of the cohort study to estimate frequency of several outcomes with the efficiency of the case–control study at measuring exposure effects. It requires a well-defined cohort of animals or herds. A subsample is taken from the full cohort to serve as a control, and detailed risk factor information is collected on these study units. Cases are then obtained from the full cohort as well as the subsample. Risk factor information for cases from outside the subsample will be collected when they become cases, and if they are from the subsample they can serve as controls before they have developed the outcome of interest.

Case–control studies can be used effectively for the study of low-incidence diseases as well as of conditions developing over a long time. They allow the investigation of preliminary causal hypotheses and are quick and relatively inexpensive, particularly in comparison with cohort studies. Their disadvantages include that they only allow the study of a single outcome and they usually cannot provide information on the disease frequency in a population. Furthermore, they are less suitable for the study of rare exposures, and data collection is reliant on the quality of past records. As discussed above, it can be very difficult to ensure an unbiased selection of the control group. Both Rothman *et al.* (2008c) and Dohoo *et al.* (2009) provide detailed information on case–control study design.

Cross-sectional study

One of the most commonly used study designs in epidemiology is the *cross-sectional study*. It is often used to obtain information about baseline characteristics of a population. In a cross-sectional study, a study group of animals from a source population is selected at one point in time. Individual animals included in the study group are examined for the presence of disease and their status with regard to risk factors (see Figure 4.4). Disease prevalence can then be estimated and compared between risk factor categories. Various random sampling strategies can be used to select the study group, including stratified, cluster and multistage sampling described in Chapter 7.

Cross-sectional studies have a number of important advantages over other observational study designs. They are useful for describing the characteristics of a population of interest, including prevalence for one or more outcomes at a particular time. The data should be based on a representative sample drawn from the population of interest (= source population). Cross-sectional studies are relatively quick to conduct and their cost is moderate. Disadvantages include that they provide only a 'snapshot in time' of the disease occurrence, and that, because of the measurement of prevalence, risk factors associated with disease risk cannot be distinguished from those linked with disease duration. It is difficult to investigate cause–effect relationships, since exposure and disease are measured at the same time. This becomes problematic for time-varying risk factors, as their effect cannot be correctly measured. It can also be difficult to obtain sufficiently large response rates, particularly with mail questionnaire studies, resulting in a potentially biased sample.

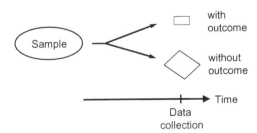

Figure 4.4   Schematic diagram of a cross-sectional study.

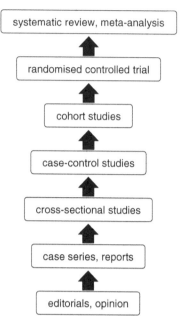

Figure 4.5 Hierarchy of evidence for cause–effect relationships derived from different study designs and information sources.

Comparison of study types

With any scientific investigation, an awareness of the limitations and advantages of particular study designs is essential during the planning, analysis and interpretation of epidemiological studies. The hierarchy of strength of evidence for cause–effect relationships provided by the different study types is shown in Figure 4.5. The best evidence can be obtained from systematic reviews, followed by an RCT which is an experimental study type and then a cohort study as the most informative observational study type. Evidence gained from editorials in scientific journals or personal opinion is least useful. Fletcher and Fletcher (2005), Cockcroft and Holmes (2003) and Greenhalgh (2006) provide further discussion of the hierarchy of scientific evidence.

5 Measuring effects

Learning objectives

After completing this chapter, you will be able to:

- Assess the strength of association between a risk factor and an outcome variable such as disease.
- Measure the impact of a risk factor on an outcome variable such as disease.

Introduction

An epidemiological study of the cause–effect relationships between potential risk factors and an outcome parameter such as disease or death usually is based on a comparison of risks or rates. *Risk factors* include any factors associated with differences in the risk of disease or mortality. Exposure to a risk factor means that an individual has, before becoming ill or having died, been affected by the risk factor. Comparison of risk requires the estimation of disease frequency (e.g. incidence rate or risk, or prevalence) for different exposure categories associated with a particular risk factor, except in the case of case–control studies where the exposure frequency is compared between different outcome, typically health status, (= case–control status) categories. The comparison can be performed by using measures either of strength of association or of potential impact. The first group involves calculation of ratios such as risk and odds ratio which measure the magnitude of the association between a risk factor and disease. They are useful for identifying risk factors, but do

Table 5.1 Structure and notation of 2×2 table to be used for calculating epidemiological measures of association

Disease status	Exposure status		Total
	Exposed	Non-exposed	
Diseased	a_1	a_0	m_1
Non-diseased	b_1	b_0	m_0
Total	n_1	n_0	n

not provide information on absolute risk. It is important to recognise that testing the statistical significance of an association between a risk factor and an outcome will not quantify the magnitude of the effect, only the likelihood that the association was due to chance, and this result will be influenced by sample size. Measures of potential impact include the risk difference and the attributable fraction. These quantify the consequences in terms of absolute risk resulting from exposure to a risk factor. They therefore give an indication of the importance of a risk factor, and can be used to predict the effect of prevention and control measures at population level. The statistical uncertainty associated with these measures of effect can be expressed by calculating confidence intervals. Chapter 6 presents the relevant mathematical calculations for risk and odds ratios, and others can be found in Morris and Gardner (2000).

The calculations of measures of effect between exposure to a risk factor and an outcome such as disease can be performed more easily after summarising the data using a 2×2 table, as presented in Table 5.1. Here, the counts in the cells identified as a_1, a_0, b_1 and b_0 represent the data as defined according to disease and exposure status. The notation is consistent with that used by Dohoo *et al.* (2009) and will be used throughout this chapter.

Measures of strength of association

Risk ratio

The risk ratio (= relative risk, cumulative incidence ratio or prevalence ratio) is usually calculated as the ratio between incidence risk of exposed and non-exposed animals (see Equation 5.1). Prevalence can only be used if the disease has a short duration and therefore prevalence can be considered to be an estimate of incidence risk. The risk ratio (RR) is interpreted as follows: the disease is RR times as likely to occur among those exposed to the suspected risk factor as among those with no such exposure. It is also possible to express the RR as a percentage, in that an RR of 1.1 would represent a 10% increase in risk, whereas an RR of 3 would be a 200% increase. RR ranges from 0 to ∞ and has no units. If RR is close to 1 (i.e. the two risks which are compared are similar and therefore the numerator and denominator values are also similar), the exposure is probably not associated with the risk of disease. If RR is greater or smaller than 1, the exposure is likely to be associated with the risk of disease, and the greater the departure from 1 the stronger the association. Values less than 1 indicate protection and those greater an increased disease risk among exposed animals. It is important to remember that RR gives no indication of absolute risk. It is a measure of relative effect, and therefore RR values can be very high even though disease risk is quite low. RR cannot be estimated in case–control studies, as these studies do not allow calculation of risks.

$$RR = (a_1/n_1)/(a_0/n_0) \tag{5.1}$$

Incidence rate ratio

The incidence rate ratio (IR) (= rate ratio or incidence density ratio) is calculated as the ratio between incidence rate estimates in exposed and non-exposed animals. It can only be obtained from studies which allow calculation of incidence rates, such as the cohort study. The IR is interpreted as the disease rate in exposed animals being IR times as high as the rate in non-exposed. Its values can range from 0 to ∞ and have no units. As with the risk ratio, if the IR value is close to 1, it is unlikely that the risk factor is associated with disease frequency. The further the value departs from unity, the more likely it is that the risk factor is associated with disease frequency. Values less than 1 indicate protection and those greater than 1 increased rates of disease in exposed animals.

Odds ratio

The odds ratio (OR) (= relative odds, cross-product ratio or approximate relative risk) is calculated as the ratio between the odds of disease in exposed animals and the odds of disease in non-exposed ones, or alternatively as the ratio of the cross-products (see Equation 5.2). The odds of disease are algebraically related to the probability or risk of disease, as they are the ratio between the probability of having the disease and the probability of not having it. In contrast to the risk ratio, the OR can be calculated for all study designs. For cohort and cross-sectional studies, the OR is interpreted as the odds of disease among exposed animals being OR times the odds of disease among non-exposed. Its meaning is therefore similar to that of the risk ratio. In an unmatched case–control study, the odds of being a case cannot be calculated, since animals were selected on the basis of case–control status. Instead, the odds of being exposed can be estimated separately for cases and controls, and their ratio is then the OR. For a pair-matched case–control study, the OR is the ratio between the counts of discordant matched pairs (i.e. the number of matched pairs where the case is exposed and the control is not, relative to the number of pairs where the opposite is true). In contrast to risk and rate ratio, the calculated OR values are the same whether the odds of disease or of non-disease are used in the calculation. The OR is an estimate of RR if the disease is rare (i.e. prevalence or incidence risk is less than 5%). In a case–control study applying a risk-based design, the OR is a good estimate of the incidence rate ratio for rare diseases. In a rate-based case–control study, the OR is a direct estimate of the incidence rate ratio. The OR can range from $-\infty$ to $+\infty$. If the OR is close to 1 (i.e. the odds for both groups are similar), there is unlikely to be an association between risk factor and disease. For an OR greater or smaller than 1, the strength of the association between the risk factor and the disease increases, and the greater the departure from 1 the stronger the potential cause–effect relationship. The advantages of the OR include that it can be obtained from all study designs, and also from logistic regression analysis.

$$OR = (a_1/b_1)/(a_0/b_0) = a_1 b_0 / a_0 b_1 \qquad (5.2)$$

Measures of impact

Risk difference

When intending to determine the amount of disease due to a risk factor, it is necessary to separate the effect of that risk factor from that of other factors that might also cause disease (sometimes called the *baseline risk*). As long as the exposed and non-exposed animals studied are similar with respect to the distribution of all other risk factors, one can assume that the baseline risk is quantified by the risk of disease in non-exposed animals. In that case, subtraction of the risk in non-exposed from the risk in exposed animals would allow quantifying the amount of disease that is likely to occur due to the risk factor (see Equation 5.3). The resulting quantity is called the *risk difference* (RD) (= attributable risk, excess risk, cumulative incidence difference or prevalence difference). If the difference between rates in exposed and non-exposed animals is calculated, the result is called an incidence rate difference. The RD is a measure of absolute risk, and is interpreted as the risk over and above the baseline risk of developing the disease being increased by RD for those individuals exposed to the risk factor. RD varies between 0 and 1, and has no units, whereas the incidence rate difference varies between $-\infty$ and $+\infty$, and has units of 1/time. If the resulting value is less than 0, the factor is protective, if it is close to 0 it has no effect and if it is greater than 1 it increases the risk of disease. Neither the risk nor the incidence rate difference can be calculated for case–control studies, since they do not generate estimates of disease frequency.

$$RD = (a_1/n_1) - (a_0/n_0) \qquad (5.3)$$

If the data have been obtained from a sample representative of the population of interest, the population attributable risk (PAR) can be calculated. It expresses the importance of the risk factor in the general population, i.e. across exposure levels. PAR can be estimated by multiplying RD by the proportion of exposed animals in the study group (see Equation 5.4).

$$PAR = RD \times (m_1/n) = (m_1/n) - (a_0/n_0) \qquad (5.4)$$

Since the RD is relatively difficult to communicate, an alternative method for interpreting it is the *number needed to treat* (NNT). This is considered to be easier to understand in a clinical context, and is interpreted as the number of (animal) patients that need to be treated with a therapy during the duration of an experimental field study in order to prevent one bad outcome. It is calculated as the inverse of the risk difference (i.e. 1/RD). When applying this parameter, it is important to take into account the follow-up period used in the study that generated it. The *number needed to harm* (NNH) can also be calculated.

Attributable fraction

The *attributable fraction* (= aetiological fraction) is a relative measure of the importance of a risk factor, and it expresses the proportion of total risk in exposed animals which is due to the risk factor. Assuming a causal effect of the risk factor, this means that the attributable fraction also represents the proportional risk reduction resulting from removing the risk factor. The calculations have to be adjusted when a risk factor is protective, in that lack of exposure has to become the effect that increases the risk (see below for discussion on vaccine efficacy). It can be calculated directly using the values for risk difference and total risk in exposed animals, or from the risk or odds ratio (see Equation 5.5). As long as the odds ratio is a good estimate of the RR in a case–control study (i.e. incidence is low), it is possible to produce an estimate of the attributable fraction also for a case–control study.

$$AF = RD/(a_1/n_1) = (RR - 1)/RR \cong (OR - 1)/OR \qquad (5.5)$$

Similarly to AF and PAR, the population-attributable fraction (PAF) quantifies the importance of a causal risk factor in the total population, rather than only the exposed animals. It is based on dividing the PAR by the disease prevalence in the study group (see Equation 5.6). It is interpreted as the probability that randomly selected animals from a group/population develop the disease as a result of the risk factor. If the proportion exposed declines in the general population, PAF also decreases, even if RR remains the same. A high PAF implies that the risk factor is important for the general animal population. PAF can also be estimated for unmatched case–control studies.

$$PAF = PAR/(m_1/n) \qquad (5.6)$$

Vaccine efficacy (= prevented fraction) is a special form of attributable fraction which stands for the proportion of disease prevented by the vaccine in vaccinated animals. It is estimated by subtracting incidence risk in vaccinated animals from incidence risk in unvaccinated animals, and dividing the resulting value by the incidence risk in unvaccinated animals.

Comparing epidemiological measures of effect

As an example data on piglet mortality and occurrence of mastitis–metritis–agalactiae complex (MMA) has been collected in a piggery with two farrowing sheds and a total of 200 sows, with equal numbers going through each shed. The design of one of the two sheds allows for easy disinfection and cleaning (= good hygiene), whereas the other shed is very difficult to clean (= poor

Table 5.2   Example calculation for risk factor comparison

		Hygiene status	
		Poor	Good
Incidence risk	Litters with deaths	0.25	0.05
	MMA	0.05	0.01
	Number of sows	100	100
	Epidemiological effect measures		
	Risk ratio	5	5
	Risk difference	0.20	0.04
	Attributable fraction	0.8	0.8

hygiene). The relevance of the different epidemiological measures can be illustrated by estimating the effect of shed hygiene as a potential risk factor affecting the incidence risk of piglet mortality (measured as occurring or not occurring on a litter basis) and MMA in sows. Summary data for 200 sows and their litters over a period of 6 months provides the information listed in Table 5.2. The numbers presented in the table indicate that the risk factor hygiene status of the shed has the same strength of association (RR = 5) for both incidence risk of piglet deaths and incidence risk of MMA. The risk difference is considerably higher for litter deaths, because they are more common. Hence, the probability of having piglet deaths in a litter given the presence of the risk factor is much higher than of having a sow with MMA. Control of the risk factor (improving the hygiene standard of the farrowing shed) will probably be justified on the basis of the economic benefits resulting from decreasing piglet mortality, but not necessarily, if it were only to control the incidence of MMA alone. The proportion of cases (litters with piglet deaths or sows with MMA) due to the presence of the risk factor (the attributable fraction) is in both cases the same.

Considering error and cause–effect

Learning objectives

After completing this chapter, you will be able to:

- Recognise the potential sources of bias in studies.
- Understand the basic concepts of estimation and statistical hypothesis testing.
- Understand the concepts of confounding and interaction.
- Describe the steps involved in the process of establishing cause–effect relationships.

Introduction

Any study will produce estimates for a parameter of interest that are affected by some degree of error, resulting in differences from the true parameter value. The types of error can be broadly classified into random and systematic error. *Random* or *chance error* is the result of taking a subset or sample of study units from the source population. It can be influenced by sample size or study design and its impact can be evaluated using statistical analysis methods. *Systematic error* or *bias* refers to non-random differences between true and estimated parameter values. It will be present in almost every study and needs to be taken into account during the design, analysis and interpretation, so that valid conclusions can be drawn. It cannot normally be quantified and therefore needs to be considered when designing a study and also when interpreting the findings. An internally valid study will allow valid conclusions about the source population, whereas external validity refers to inferences about the target population. Both Dohoo *et al.* (2009) and Rothman *et al.* (2008a) provide detailed discussions on validity.

Systematic error

Any process during a scientific study which results in systematic (non-random) departure of the observed from the true values is called systematic error or bias. There are three main types of bias: selection, information and confounding bias.

Selection bias is largely affected by study design, particularly by the selection process of the study units. It refers to differences between the study group and source population which lead to a biased observed relationship between risk factors and the outcome of interest. It can be the result of differences in the selection of study subgroups. For example, the selection of the control group in a case–control study is often subject to selection bias, particularly if the cases have been obtained from a hospital referral population and whenever it is not possible to identify the source population of the cases. Non-response in a mail questionnaire survey may result in bias, if responders are systematically different from non-responders. In a study of controversial animal husbandry practices, for example, users of these practices may be more likely to not respond. In cohort studies, the likelihood of loss to follow-up could be associated with a risk factor and thereby lead to selection bias.

Information bias is the result of incorrect measurement of risk factor and/ or disease status. In case of categorical-type variables such as breed it is called *misclassification bias* and for continuous-scale variables such as body weight it is called *measurement error*. Poor accuracy of a diagnostic test will lead to misclassification, as will inaccurate responses to questionnaires, e.g. as a result of poor recall.

Confounding bias has also been called the mixing of effects of different risk factors. It means that a risk factor of interest is associated with the outcome as well as with other risk factors, some of which may have been measured and some not. The observed effect of a particular risk factor may therefore wholly or partially represent the effect of these other factors on the outcome. The other factor(s) in such a case would be the confounder(s). Confounding can be controlled either during study design through methods such as matching or during the statistical analysis through stratification or multivariable adjustment. When using stratified data analyses to test for the presence of confounding, the association between exposure and outcome is assessed in separate (= stratified) analyses for each level of the hypothesised

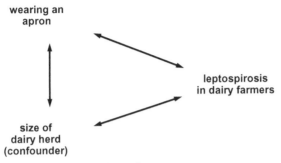

Figure 6.1 Example of confounding relationship.

confounding factor. If the strength of the association between exposure and outcome weakens after controlling for the confounder, meaning the risk ratios for each of the strata are closer to unity than the so-called crude risk ratio, then there is a potential risk for confounding. As an example for a confounding relationship, during the analysis of data from a study of leptospirosis in dairy farm workers in New Zealand the investigators discovered that wearing an apron during milking was associated with an increased risk of contracting leptospirosis (Mackintosh *et al.* 1980). Naive interpretation of the data could therefore have resulted in the conclusion that if dairy farm workers wanted to reduce the risk of leptospirosis infection they should not wear an apron during milking. But before publicising this result, the investigators found that the risk of infection seemed to increase with herd size, and – more importantly – farmers with larger herds were found to be more likely to wear aprons during milking than farmers with smaller herds (see Figure 6.1). The authors concluded that the apparent association between wearing an apron and leptospirosis infection was in reality due to the confounding of the true effect of herd size.

Random error

General principles

Random or *chance error* is any variability in the data that cannot be explained. It can be influenced by sample size and study design, and estimated using statistical analysis methods. An increase in sample size will result in reduced random error, assuming that the selection of study units was done randomly. If specific factors are known to increase random variation, the study design can be tailored so that this variation can be controlled during the selection process of the study units. The impact of chance can be evaluated either through estimation or by statistical hypothesis testing. Both approaches are discussed below. As a very brief background on sampling theory, the central

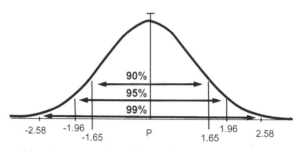

Figure 6.2 Central limit theorem and confidence limits.

limit theorem is the basis of the variance estimates calculated for probability sampling data. The central limit theorem states that, given large sample sizes, the distribution of sample means or proportions tends to be normal. Using this concept, confidence intervals can be calculated with 90% of estimates ranging between −1.65 and +1.65 standard errors from the mean, 95% between −1.96 and +1.96 standard errors and 99% between −2.58 and +2.58 standard errors (see Figure 6.2).

Estimation

Estimation implies that an epidemiological quantity such as a disease frequency or an effect measure is being quantified, together with the degree of precision it has been measured with. If the effect is presented as a single value, it is called a *point estimate* and the precision can be expressed using a confidence interval. The width of the confidence interval determines whether precision is low or high. Usually confidence intervals are defined based on a 90, 95 or 99% confidence level. As an example, the interpretation of a 95% confidence interval for a particular parameter is that if one were to conduct the same study 100 times and estimate a 95% confidence interval for the parameter of interest for each of them, then about 95 of the 100 confidence intervals will include the true value of the estimate of interest. Note that this assumes the underlying statistical model is appropriate and that confounding bias is absent. If a 95% confidence interval includes the null value for an epidemiological measure of effect, such as 1 for the odds ratio or risk ratio, it indicates that it is not statistically different from the null value.

Statistical hypothesis testing

Statistical hypothesis testing involves determining whether an observed difference is statistically significant on the basis of testing whether a particular hypothesis can be rejected or not. Usually it concerns a null hypothesis indicating that there is no association between two factors in the population from which the sample used in this analysis was selected. This is quite important, since while there may be a difference in the sample or study group, the important question is whether there is one in the target or source population. It is important to recognise that statistical hypothesis testing does not assess whether the null hypothesis or any hypothesis is correct or false. Instead, it tests if the null hypothesis can be rejected, which in turn leads to the interpretation that a result (usually an association between two factors) is statistically significant. If it cannot be rejected, the result of the analysis is not statistically significant. The decision on whether the null hypothesis can be rejected or not is based on the p-value, which quantifies the probability that the observed association is the result of random variation, and this value is often set to a level of 0.05. As an example, a χ^2-squared test could be used to test the difference in incidence risk between animals exposed and not exposed to a risk factor for statistical significance. If the χ^2 value is greater than 3.84, the associated p-value is less than 0.05. This p-value can be interpreted as follows using frequentist statistical theory. It is assumed that the study is repeated 100 times; each time the study units are randomly selected from the source population and the value for the test statistic (e.g. χ^2 value) is calculated. In the case of the above example, if there was no association between the two factors (= the null hypothesis), one would expect the observed difference between the two proportions to occur just due to chance variation less than 5 times out of the 100 samples taken from the source population. Assuming that one accepts $p \leq 0.05$ as a decision criterion for statistical significance, it can be concluded for this hypothetical example that there is a statistically significant association between risk factor and disease incidence risk. Clearly, just reporting statistical significance on the basis of whether a test statistic was above or below a cut-off (e.g. $\chi^2 = 3.84$ for $p < 0.05$) is a very crude way of summarising the result of the analysis. Since the actual p-value for the test statistic may be very near or far away from that cut-off, it is recommended that the actual p-values are reported. But even if this is done, the p-value does not allow differentiation between the strength and direction of an effect and its statistical precision. It is also important to note that none of these quantities describes clinical relevance. As an example, if a treatment is cheap and has no clinical side effects, but may result in improved prognosis for a disease seriously compromising the animal's welfare, a p-value as high as 0.10 or more may be sufficient for the clinician to apply the treatment. On the other hand, if the treatment has serious clinical side effects and is expensive, a p-value much less than 0.05 may be desirable before the treatment is applied in a particular animal.

The following concepts are important for statistical hypothesis testing. Firstly, as discussed above there is a null hypothesis (H_0) which is to be tested with respect to whether it can be rejected or not in favour of an alternative hypothesis (H_1). Then there is chance variation (= random error) which can result in making either a type I or type II error (see Figure 6.3). A type I error (= α-error or false positive) refers to incorrectly rejecting the null hypothesis.

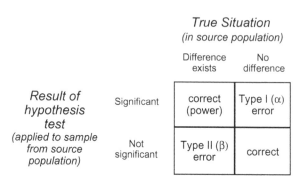

Figure 6.3 Correct decisions and errors in statistical hypothesis testing.

The *p*-value quantifies the likelihood of a type I error. In a type II error (= β-error or false negative), the null hypothesis is false but has not been rejected. *Statistical power* (calculated as 1 – type II error) denotes the probability that a study will find a statistical difference if it does in fact exist. Note that there are small-sample (= exact) and large-sample (= asymptotic) methods for calculating the above probabilities. Small-sample methods have become more accessible for use in epidemiological analysis as a result of the increased computational power available for performing the much more complex calculations. They lead to Monte-Carlo or exact *p*-values. Large-sample statistics are still most commonly used, but it needs to be kept in mind that they are based on the assumption of large sample sizes. Large-sample statistical analysis is based on using the observed data to calculate the value for the appropriate test statistic (e.g. χ^2 test). The probability of the occurrence of this value assuming that there is no association is then calculated from a theoretical distribution appropriate for the particular statistical test (e.g. χ^2, t or F).

Comparing estimation and statistical hypothesis testing

The following hypothetical example explores the difference between statistical hypothesis testing and estimation. The association or relationship between two breed groups as a risk factor and disease status is being assessed. The study was conducted as a 1-year cohort study with 100 animals in each exposure category. At the end of the study, the incidence risk was 0.50 for breed A and 0.30 for breed B. Using a 2 × 2 table, a χ^2 value of 8.33 with 1 degree of freedom and an associated *p*-value of 0.004 can be calculated (see Table 6.1). If we had decided on a cut-off of $p < 0.05$, we can conclude that the null hypothesis of the risk of infection in this population being independent of breed can be rejected. Therefore, the two variables are statistically significantly associated. Hence, the disease incidence is different between the two breeds. And since one proportion is smaller than the other, we can also conclude that

Table 6.1 Comparison of risk of infection between breeds

Infection status	Breed	
	A	B
Positive	50	30
Negative	50	70
Incidence risk (per year)	0.50	0.30

the risk is higher for breed A than for breed B. Given that the actual p-value is available, more information about the relationship can be obtained. A p-value of 0.004 indicates that the observed difference between the two proportions would be expected to occur due to chance variation alone less than 4 times in 1000 samples from a source population assumed to have no difference between breeds. This now indicates that it is indeed very unlikely for this difference to be obtained if there is no association between breed and disease status. But still, neither stating statistical significance nor reporting actual p-values will distinguish between effect sizes and precision. This is where estimation is useful. In this example, we could obtain a point estimate of the risk ratio which is calculated from the ratio of the two incidence risks as 1.7. The statistical precision of the risk ratio value of 1.7 can be expressed through the 95% confidence interval from 1.16 to 2.38. This clearly demonstrates the value of estimation, in that the indication of the strength and direction of the effect (= risk ratio of 1.7) is clearly separated from its precision (= true value likely to vary between 1.16 and 2.38). A more detailed discussion of these concepts can be found in Rothman *et al.* (2008b).

Mathematical formulas for confidence interval calculation of proportions and ratio effect measures

The calculation of confidence intervals for proportions, such as incidence risk and prevalence, is based on the point estimate p itself and the sample size n. This information is then used to calculate the standard error SE, as shown in Equation 6.1:

$$SE = \sqrt{[p(1-p)/n]} \qquad (6.1)$$

where SE is the standard error of observed proportion, p is the observed proportion and n is sample size.

The SE is then combined with the point estimate p to calculate the upper and lower confidence limits CL as shown in Equation 6.2. The value for Z reflects the desired confidence level, and values for z of 1.65, 1.96 and 2.58 represent 90%, 95% and 99% confidence levels, respectively.

$$CL = p \pm Z \times SE \tag{6.2}$$

where CL denotes confidence limits (upper and lower), Z is the Z-value reflecting the desired level of confidence, p is the observed proportion and SE its standard error.

As an example, if the observed prevalence of positive tuberculin tests is 10% among 80 cattle tested, the lower and upper 95% confidence limits can be calculated as follows:

$$CL_{lower} = 0.1 - 1.96 \times \sqrt{\{([0.1 \times (1 - 0.1)]/80\}} = 0.03$$

$$CL_{upper} = 0.1 + 1.96 \times \sqrt{\{([0.1 \times (1 - 0.1)]/80\}} = 0.17$$

Based on the above calculations, the 95% confidence interval for the observed prevalence of 10% in this group of 75 cattle ranges from 0.03 to 0.17. Note that this confidence interval calculation is based on the Wald normal approximation which is valid for large sample sizes. The more complex calculations for obtaining exact estimates of the confidence limits are accessible via online tools such as OpenEpi (www.openepi.org), or standalone public domain software, such as WinEpiscope (www.clive.ed.ac.uk/winepiscope), EpiInfo (www.cdc.gov/epiinfo/) or Win-PEPI (www.brixtonhealth.com).

Confidence intervals for ratio effect measures such as risk or odds ratio are calculated similarly to those for proportions, in that a point estimate is combined with an estimate of error, in this case variance. The calculations have to be performed on a log scale, and the variance of $\ln RR$ and $\ln OR$ can be obtained using a first-order Taylor series approximation. The relevant formulas are shown in Equations 6.3 and 6.4, respectively:

$$var(\ln PR) = 1/a_1 + 1/n_1 + 1/a_0 + 1/n_0 \tag{6.3}$$

where var($\ln RR$) is the variance of the log scale risk ratio point estimate, a_1 is the number of exposed animals with disease, n_1 is the total number of exposed animals, a_0 is the number of non-exposed animals with disease and n_0 is the total number of non-exposed animals.

$$var(\ln OR) = 1/a_1 + 1/a_0 + 1/b_1 + 1/b_0 \tag{6.4}$$

where var($\ln OR$) is the variance of the log scale odds ratio point estimate, a_1 is the number of exposed animals with disease, a_0 is the number of non-exposed animals with disease, b_1 is the number of exposed animals without disease and b_0 is the number of non-exposed animals without disease.

The formula for the calculation of the confidence interval for a ratio point estimate θ is shown in Equation 6.5.

$$CL = \theta \times \exp\left\{\pm Z \sqrt{[\mathrm{var}(\ln \theta)]}\right\} \qquad (6.5)$$

where CL denotes confidence limits (upper and lower), Z is the Z-value reflecting the desired level of confidence and θ is the ratio point estimate.

More complete information about the mathematical formulas for various statistical tests and calculation of confidence interval effect estimates is available in most statistics and epidemiology textbooks. Altman *et al.* (2000) provide example confidence interval calculations for many epidemiological outcome parameters. The calculations for relevant epidemiological parameters can also be performed using online tools, mentioned above.

Interaction or effect modification

In most biological systems, multiple factors will influence the risk of disease occurrence. Any estimation of effects becomes more difficult if these factors are not independent of each other, meaning that the effect of one factor depends on the level of another. This relationship is called *interaction* or *effect modification*. It reflects a biological property of the joint effect of these factors and can manifest itself as either synergism or antagonism. Statistical interaction is considered to be present when the combined effect of variables on an outcome measure differs from the sum of the individual effects at a defined scale. There is therefore a multiplicative rather than additive relationship between the effects of the variables. If statistical interaction refers to causal effects, it implies biological interaction. But biological interaction may still be present even if statistical interaction cannot be demonstrated.

Stratified analysis can be used to assess epidemiological data for the presence of interaction. If there is no interaction, stratum-specific risk or odds ratios should be equal. Figure 6.4a presents an example of two factors which do not interact. This becomes evident after stratifying on factor 1 (= holding this factor constant), as the stratum-specific risk ratio estimates are both 2. An example of interaction between two risk factors is shown in Figure 6.4b. These data relate to a cohort study in cows aimed at determining risk factors associated with abortion risk. During the 1-year study period, all cows were assessed serologically for *Neospora caninum* and bovine virus diarrhoea (BVD) infection status as potential risk factors. To test for possible statistical interaction between these two risk factors, the data were stratified by *Neospora* infection

(a)

Factor A	Factor B	Incidence risk	Risk ratio (within stratum)	Risk ratio (compared with both factors being absent)
present	present	0.16	2	8
present	absent	0.08	2	4
absent	present	0.04	2	2
absent	absent	0.02	2	reference

equal RRs

(b)

Abortion

Neospora ELISA	BVD ELISA	yes	no	Incidence risk	Risk ratio (within stratum)	Risk ratio (compared with both factors being absent)
positive	positive	45	10	0.82	3.27	3.68
positive	negative	2	6	0.25	3.27	1.13
negative	positive	21	58	0.27	1.20	1.20
negative	negative	8	28	0.22	1.20	reference

different RRs

Figure 6.4 Examples without (a) and with (b) statistical interaction.

status. The resulting stratum-specific risk ratio estimates quantifying the effect of BVD serology status on abortion incidence risk in cows vary substantially between the two strata. It suggests that cows positive to both of the infectious organisms were more than three times as likely to abort as those that were positive to only one of them. Assuming that there was no important bias involved, this finding indicates that there is a statistical interaction relationship. Further studies would be necessary to assess the possible presence of a biological interaction between these two risk factors.

A Venn diagram is a useful method for visually examining interaction relationships between several risk factors. Figure 6.5 presents an example of such a diagram based on the above epidemiological field study of potential risk factors for bovine abortion. Age group (age ≤ 3 years) has been added as a third risk factor to BVD and *Neospora* serological status. The diagram shows the risk ratio values for different combinations of the three risk factors compared with a reference group of cows which are older than 3 years and serologically negative for both BVD and *Neospora*. The diagram indicates that the risk for cows to abort is 4.1 times as high if they are both BVD positive and ≤3 years of age. This suggests that there is also a statistical interaction

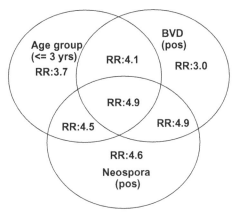

Figure 6.5 Venn diagram relationships between three risk factors for a study on abortion in cows.

between these two factors since they each by themselves have lower risk ratios. The combination of being ≤3 years and positive for both serological tests does not increase the risk ratio beyond the value already reached for animals which are positive to both tests. In summary, there does not appear to be an interaction between all three factors, although this finding needs to be interpreted carefully as the number of animals in the various strata used for this example was quite small.

From association to cause and effect

So far, the effects of random and systematic error have been discussed separately. The process of assessing a potential cause–effect relationship between a risk factor with two exposure categories and an outcome variable of interest such as infection status of an animal can be structured as described in the flowchart shown in Figure 6.6. It is assumed that the data have already been collected and are now being analysed. As a first step the observed disease frequencies are calculated for each exposure group and then compared between the groups of exposed and non-exposed. An apparent association between the potential risk factor and disease status is considered to be present on the basis of, say, there being a higher incidence risk of the disease among animals exposed to the risk factor than in those not exposed. If this is indeed the case, the question arises whether there is one in the source population from which the study group was selected and in the target population. The data should first be assessed for bias in the selection of the animals studied and accuracy of the information about risk factor or disease status. If it has been concluded that there is little bias, the next step is to assess the likelihood that the observed

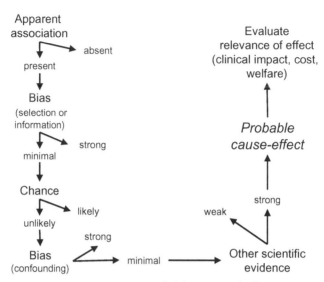

Figure 6.6   From apparent association to probable cause and effect.

difference was due to random or chance error using an appropriate statistical test. If the statistical analysis results in a low p-value, say 0.01, it is unlikely that the observed difference between the incidence risks is due to chance. As discussed above, one would preferably calculate a point estimate of the effect of interest, the risk ratio in this case, and its 95% confidence interval. If the confidence interval does not include a risk ratio of 1, then this is a statistically significant effect. But even at this stage of the analysis, apart from there still being the possibility of chance error (although only a small chance) it is still possible that the statistical association between the risk factor and the disease status is due to some other unmeasured factor which is confounded with the evaluated risk factor, thereby indicating presence of confounding bias. Even if confounding bias is believed to be minimal, but the current study is the only one that has come up with this statistical association, the result still only represents weak evidence of cause and effect. Further scientific evidence is required before a cause–effect relationship can be considered as being probable. And finally, if further evidence indeed exists which suggests the presence of a probable cause–effect relationship, it may be that the effect is of limited clinical relevance with respect to its magnitude, or in case of a treatment its application may be too costly, have adverse side effects or other adverse welfare implications.

Sampling of animal populations

Learning objectives

After completing this chapter, you will be able to:

- Identify, define and differentiate the terms related to sampling methodology.
- Give advantages and disadvantages of each sampling method.
- Select the appropriate sampling strategy for a particular situation.

Introduction

An epidemiological analysis involves working with a set of observations that has been collected about a population of interest. It is important to be clear about the purpose of the results of the analysis. Usually, the inferences are about specific attributes of or relationships within an aggregate or population of individual animals or herds called the *population of interest* or *target population*. As discussed in Chapter 4, a *descriptive study* may be aimed at proving that disease is not present, detecting presence of disease or establishing the level of disease occurrence. Alternatively, its objective could be to describe levels of milk production in a population of dairy cattle or more generally provide a descriptive analysis of an animal production system. An *analytical study* will be conducted to investigate cause–effect relationships between risk factors and outcome variables, such as disease.

The data to be used for epidemiological analysis need to be evaluated with respect to completeness, validity and representativeness. They might be based on existing data or on an ongoing data collection process; or data collection may be tailored for the purposes of a specific epidemiological study. Existing data include, for example, observations made during past studies or a census, as well as ongoing data collection such as laboratory submissions, disease surveillance programmes, industry- or farm/bureau-based data recording systems and abattoirs. An awareness of the selection or information bias associated with these data sources is essential. For example, laboratory submissions are a useful mechanism for detecting disease, and they can become the basis of case series and case–control studies. But they are usually inadequate for prevalence estimation, because both the numerator and denominator are likely to be strongly affected by selection bias.

If the observations are made on every animal in the population of interest, the data collection process is called a *census*. If it is restricted to a subset of that population, it is called a *sample* or study group. The latter has the advantage over the census that results can be obtained more quickly. Data from a sample or study group is also less expensive to collect than a census, and sample results may even be more accurate as it is possible to make more efficient use of resources (e.g. better training of data collectors or use of more expensive diagnostic tests). In addition, random or probability samples result in probability estimates which allow inferences to be used for other populations. Often involvement of the whole population, as is necessary for a census, may not be possible for logistic or administrative reasons, so that sampling becomes the method of choice. A census should only be affected by information bias, although there is often also some selection bias due to non-response. Also, given that a census provides a snapshot of the population of interest at a certain point in time, it can be looked at as a single sample of many possible samples that could be taken over a time period. Samples will be affected by both selection and information bias, as well as sampling error.

The following terminology is of relevance when discussing the sampling process (see Figure 7.1). There is usually a *target population* to which study results are to be extrapolated depending on their external validity. The specification of the target population and its relationship to the source population often has to be based on judgement. The *source population* represents the immediate population for which the study conclusions are to be used, and from which a subset is to be selected. The *sampling frame* lists all sampling units in the source population, and is an important requirement for probability sampling, specifically when using simple random sampling. *Sampling units* are the individual members of the sampling frame, e.g. individual herds or animals. The *study group* or *sample* consists of the subset of members of the source population from which observations are made. *Internal validity* describes the

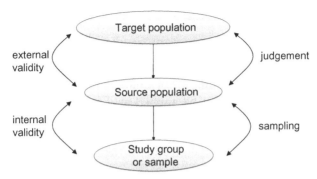

Figure 7.1 Hierarchy of the sampling process.

relationship between study and source population, whereas *external validity* refers to the relationship between source and target populations. *Sample units* are the individual members of the study group. The term *study unit* is often also applied to the sample unit, but with some sampling strategies the sample units may be different from the study units. Study units should be the elements of the study group from which measurements are taken. The sampling fraction is calculated as the ratio between the size of study group and source populations.

Probability or non-probability sampling

The aim of the sampling process is to draw a sample that is a true representation of the source and ideally the target population and which leads to estimates of population characteristics of an acceptable precision or accuracy. Samples can be selected as probability or non-probability samples. With non-probability sampling the investigator can choose the sample using three different approaches. A *convenience sample* involves taking the most easily obtainable observations, and a *purposive sample* targets specific risk groups. With a *judgement sample* the investigator makes a deliberate subjective choice to selecting what they regard to be a 'representative sample'. The main disadvantage of the non-probability sampling approach is that 'representativeness' cannot be quantified. Probability or *random sampling* requires random selection of the sample. The assumption behind the procedure is that any of the possible samples from the source population has the same chance of being selected. This means that each animal has an equal probability of selection and an animal's selection does not depend on others being selected. In practical terms there are different methods for performing random sampling, including drawing numbers from a hat, or using random numbers generated by a computer or from a random number table.

Random sampling strategies

Probability or random sampling can be applied to the individual animal or the group as the sampling unit. In the case of the former, simple random, systematic or stratified sampling are available. With cluster and multistage sampling, random selection can be applied at different levels of aggregation, and at least one of the sampling units has to be a group, such as an administrative district or a herd. The sample units resulting from these selection strategies may be a higher level aggregate of the study units.

Simple random sampling

From a statistician's perspective, simple random sampling is the optimal method for selecting observations from a population. Among its advantages is that it is based on a theoretically relatively simple concept. More importantly, the statistical theory behind standard methods of calculation of sample size and variation of sample estimates is based on the assumption that simple random sampling has been used. If other sampling methods have been used, estimates of variation may be incorrect, and therefore more complex methods of variance calculation need to be applied. The disadvantages include that simple random sampling requires a sampling frame which is often not available with animal populations. Furthermore, if there is large variation in a source population with respect to a parameter such as prevalence, very large sample sizes may be required to obtain sufficiently precise sample estimates of prevalence.

As an example, the study objective may be to determine the prevalence of *Brucella abortus* infection at the herd level in a district. Assuming that there are 1000 herds and a sample of 100 is required, the herds could be numbered from 1 to 1000. Then 100 different numbers between 1 and 1000 could be generated randomly by a computer and the herds corresponding to these numbers would represent a simple random sample.

Systematic random sampling

Systematic random sampling does not require a sampling frame, but all sample units need to be available, and they should be subject to some sort of sequence (e.g. dairy cows coming into a milking yard). The study units are selected at fixed intervals along that sequence. This sampling interval will be calculated by dividing the size of the study group with the sample size. The first animal will be selected by drawing a random number between 1 and the numeric value of the sampling interval. The advantages of this method are that it does not require a sampling frame and it is very easy to apply under field conditions. It has the disadvantage that it can introduce selection bias, if the characteristic measured is related to the sampling interval, such as when the sampling interval is associated with seasonal or behavioural effects. Given that no random sampling is involved, it is strictly speaking not possible to calculate valid variance estimates. In practice simple random sampling estimators are used, as the level of bias in the estimates is usually considered to be acceptable.

As an example, one could conduct a survey in relation to cat feeding habits among cat owners visiting a veterinary practice. Only 3 days are available for data collection. Having predefined a required sample size of 30, the typical number of cat owners visiting the practice per day can be used to calculate the sampling interval. If 50 cat owners visit the practice on average per day, the total source population over 3 days will be about 150, resulting in a sampling interval of 5. The first cat owner to be interviewed would be randomly selected, using a random number between 1 and 5. From then on, the sampling interval of 5 will be used to select the other owners comprising the sample.

Stratified random sampling

In a stratified random sample, the source population is first divided into strata based on factors that are known to affect the outcome. Within each of the strata, simple or systematic sampling is then used for selecting the sample units. If a known factor causes significant variation in the outcome variable, but is not the target of the analysis, this stratified sampling is an effective method for reducing variance in the overall parameter estimate of interest. For example, in the case of milk production in a population of dairy cows consisting of Jersey and Holstein breeds, sampling variation of estimates will be substantial, largely due to genetic differences affecting milk volume of the two breeds. Stratification on breed will allow reducing the overall variation of the milk production estimate to be obtained from the sample. In other words, for stratified sampling to be effective, the elements within the strata should be homogeneous with respect to the parameters of interest, but variance between the strata should be large. Allocation of individuals to the different strata can be in equal numbers (same n per stratum) or proportional (same n/N per stratum). The latter is used if it is necessary to ensure that the study group has the same proportional distribution of observations across the strata as the source population. Stratified sampling will also allow easy access to information about the subpopulations represented by the strata, although any stratum-specific parameter estimates will be less precise than the ones for the total population because of the smaller sample size. Disadvantages are that the status of the sample units with respect to the stratification factor needs to be known and more complex methods are required to obtain sample sizes and variance estimates.

As an example, when determining the prevalence of cattle herds infected with bovine brucellosis it may be of relevance to have the same herd size distribution in the study group comprising 100 herds as in the source popula-tion of 2000. Assuming that in the source population 20% have more than 200 adult cattle, 50% between 50 and 200, and 30% less than 50, these strata can be used to randomly select from within each of the strata 20 of the 400 large herds, 50 of the 1000 mid-size and 30 of the 600 small ones. If simple random sampling had been used, it is likely that very few large and small herds would have been selected, and these herd size categories therefore would have had little weight in the analysis.

Cluster sampling

Cluster sampling is one of the two random sampling techniques where each of the sample units is an aggregate of study units (e.g. districts, herds, litters). Typically, the individual still remains the unit of interest, e.g. its disease status, but the sample unit becomes a grouping of individual animals such as the herd they belong to. All elements within each randomly selected group are then included in the sample. This technique has the advantage that it only requires a sampling frame for the groups, but not for the members within the groups. The groups or clusters can represent natural groupings such as litters or herds, or they can be based on artificial groupings such as geographic areas or administrative units. This results in a further advantage in that to achieve a certain sample size of study units, a smaller number of sample units (i.e. clus-ters) needs to be visited. If the study units had instead been selected using simple random sampling, it would have required extensive travelling to access all study units. The random selection of the clusters as the sample units can be performed using simple, systematic or stratified random sampling. Cluster sampling assumes that the elements within the clusters are heterogeneous with respect to the parameter of interest (unlike stratified sampling). A disadvantage of cluster sampling is that it will often lead to an increased sampling variance, in accordance with the saying that 'birds of a feather flock together'. Assuming that the source population consists of cows within an administrative district and the prevalence of bovine virus diarrhoea (BVD) is to be measured, with an infectious disease such as BVD the presence of an infected animal within a herd usually means that there are also others that are infected, i.e. there is dependence with respect to infection status between the animals within herds. Therefore, if a relatively small number of herds (= clusters) has been selected, examining all cows from the selected herds will not allow appropriate repre-sentation of variability in BVD infection status at the individual animal level in the source population, and may indeed lead to an underestimate of vari-ability. This means that with data collected on the basis of cluster sampling, the variance of estimated population parameters is strongly influenced by the number of clusters, and not so much by the number of animals in the study group (i.e. the sample). In such a situation, the sample size calculations and any population parameter precision estimates should be adjusted for dependence within clusters.

An example for an application of cluster sampling is a study where the prevalence of respiratory disease is to be determined in slaughter pigs in a population associated with a particular abattoir. The clusters in this instance could be slaughter days at the abattoir, where on the randomly selected days all pigs coming for slaughter would be examined for presence of lesions indicative of respiratory disease. The advantage would be that the investigator would only have to visit the abattoir on a relatively small number of days. The disadvantage is that pigs arriving at the abattoir will probably arrive in groups from a relatively small set of farms, and there will therefore be some dependence within these groups with respect to respiratory disease risk.

Multistage sampling

Multistage sampling extends cluster sampling by using random sampling at different hierarchical levels of aggregation of the sample units. It is frequently applied as two-stage cluster sampling, where, for example, herds are randomly selected as *primary sampling units* (PSU) and within each of the selected herds animals are randomly selected as *secondary sampling units* (SSU). The key advantage of multistage sampling is that it can be used if no sampling frame is available for the sample units. As an example of two-stage cluster sampling, after the PSUs such as the herds have been randomly selected, a sampling frame for the SSUs, say the dairy cows within each selected herd, can be established at the herd visits. Another advantage of multistage compared with simple random sampling is that the ratio between the number of PSUs and SSUs can be determined taking into consideration cost and/or variability between and within PSUs. If the within-PSU variation is high relative to between-PSUs variation, a smaller number of PSUs can be selected, and more SSUs within each PSU. The cost of travel can be controlled by decreasing the number of PSUs. A disadvantage of multistage sampling is that due to dependence amongst SSUs within PSUs a larger sample size may be required to achieve the same precision as for simple random sampling. Furthermore, more complex statistical calculation methods need to be used for calculating sample sizes and quantifying variation of the parameter estimates.

Comparison of main sampling strategies

The main sampling methods are compared in Table 7.1 with respect to the population characteristics and the population types for which a particular approach is most useful. For many applications, different sampling strategies may be combined for best effect, such as in the case of the sampling strategy required under the Office International des Epizooties' pathway to declaration

Table 7.1 Comparison of main sampling strategies

Population characteristics	Example	Appropriate sampling strategy
Homogeneous	Cattle on farm; sampled to determine tuberculosis prevalence	Simple random
Definite strata, but homogeneous within strata	Farm with 2 different dairy breeds and with similar numbers of each; sampled to determine milk production	Stratified
Definite strata, each stratum has proportionate ratio of number of members relative to total	Farm with 2 different dairy breeds, but very different numbers of each; sampled to determine milk production	Proportional stratified
Groups with similar characteristics, but heterogeneous within group	Veterinary laboratories in country equipped according to standard; wide variation between samples submitted to each; sampled to determine proportion of contaminated tissue samples	Cluster
No sampling frame for units of interest	Cattle in region; sampled to determine tuberculosis prevalence	Multistage

of freedom from infection with the rinderpest virus (OIE Terrestrial Animal Health Code 2008, Article 8.13.22). Here, a country first has to be divided into strata according to disease risk, and then multistage sampling is to be conducted within each stratum. At the same time, random sampling should be conducted in purposively selected high risk areas.

Data analysis taking account of sampling strategy

As mentioned for the sampling approaches presented above, standard methods of statistical analysis assume that the data to be analysed have been collected using simple random sampling. If this is not the case, adjustments need to be made in order to obtain unbiased estimates of population parameters. The main effects to take into account are stratification, clustering and the use of sampling weights. The *design effect* quantifies the impact of the sampling strategy on the precision of the population estimates, and is calculated as the ratio between the variance obtained under a particular sampling strategy and that to be expected with simple random sampling. Appropriately applied stratification should result in a design effect of less than 1, whereas cluster sampling will have a design effect greater than 1. In case of non-proportional stratification, sampling weights may have been applied, in that the chance of individual animals being selected varies between strata. In this case, the selection probability of an animal needs to be calculated for each stratum, and then each animal observation has to be re-weighted according to the inverse of the sampling weight when calculating overall population parameters (see Dohoo *et al.* 2009 for further details). If a stratified, cluster or multistage sampling approach has been used, complex mathematical procedures need to be applied that require the use of specialised computer software.

Miscellaneous sampling strategies

The methods discussed in detail above are most commonly used in epidemiological research, but there are several other techniques that should be mentioned. A number of them have been developed in social science or ecological research, and they usually require the use of mathematically complex variance adjustments in the data analysis.

In *post-stratification*, information on the strata was not available before the study, but it is one of the study objectives to obtain precise parameter estimates for each stratum. Here, a simple random sample has to be used, and the data are stratified for the analysis.

Quota sampling refers to the situation where a population is divided into strata, but no sampling frame is available. Selection of sample units then occurs until a predefined quota is achieved within each stratum.

With *adaptive sampling*, the aim is to maximise detection of units of interest with rare attributes which would be absent or under-represented in the sample if simple random sampling was used. The approach implies that selection of further sample units is redirected depending on the attributes of already selected sample units (e.g. being in the same neighbourhood, having had contact, genetic similarity). As an example, a study might be conducted to identify farmers trading a particular type of animal breed, and characterise the network linking them. Here, the researcher may start with a number of known farmers, and then identify further members of the sample by asking each farmer about their contacts, which will then be asked by their contacts, and so on. This approach is called *snowball sampling*. Thompson and Collins (2002) discuss a number of other applications of adaptive sampling designs. *Double* or *two-phase sampling* can be applied in different ways. A simple random sample may be used to inform a second study phase with respect to relevant strata or cases and controls. Alternatively, a mail questionnaire study may be conducted, and non-responders may become the subject of the second phase of the study.

Lot quality assurance sampling (LQAS) has been developed in the context of industrial quality control. Its principle is that a certain sample size is collected from a population or stratum, and if a threshold number of units sampled show a certain characteristic (e.g. farms that do not vaccinate) then the population or stratum is considered to fail a quality decision criterion (e.g. adequate vaccination coverage).

Capture–mark–recapture sampling was originally developed for wild animal population research. It has more recently been applied in epidemiological research for obtaining more accurate population counts for open populations, and involves combining data from different overlapping data sources. Thompson (2002) and Levy and Lemeshow (2008) provide detailed information about the above sampling approaches.

Sample size calculation

Deciding the necessary sample size is crucial to any epidemiological study. The methods for calculating sample size can be broadly grouped into those for studies estimating a population parameter such as disease prevalence or average body weight and those aimed at describing effects or differences within a population. There are several factors to take into consideration when defining sample size. These are the expected variation of the variable of interest in the population, the required precision, the desired level of confidence, the design effect and, for analytical studies, the statistical power. As pointed out by Rothman *et al.* (2008b), statistical sample size calculations are only one component of the factors to consider when deciding on the size of a study. Others are the costs of the study and the often not quantifiable benefits which may potentially be derived from its findings.

The *expected variation* refers to how variable the parameter of interest is in the source population. Variability for proportions is calculated as the product of $p \times (1 - p)$, as shown in Table 7.2. Using prevalence as an example, variability will be highest for prevalence values of 0.5. This is because for this value, there is an equal chance of sampling units being diseased or non-

Table 7.2 Calculation of variability for proportions

p	$p \times (1 - p)$
0.9	0.09
0.7	0.21
0.5	0.25
0.3	0.21
0.1	0.09

diseased. If several random samples of the same size are then taken from the same source population, it will result in more variation among prevalence estimates than if prevalence had been a lower or higher value. If prevalence is low, there are too few diseased animals in the source population for there to be large variation between sample estimates. The expected variance of continuous scale parameters such as body weight is easier to define when considered in terms of standard deviation. If we can estimate the range within which 95% of values will be around the mean, this represents 4 standard deviations. A rough estimate of the variance can be calculated by dividing the range by 4 and squaring the resulting value.

The *desired precision* range of the estimate indicates how far the estimate obtained from the sample can be from the true value in the source population. Its value should be based on the decision that will be influenced by the estimate obtained from the study. For example, if one expects disease prevalence to be 30% in the population of interest, the chance of the estimate obtained from a sample of that population being close to that value will increase with sample size. In this case, it may not matter whether the sample estimate is any value between 25% and 35%, but if it was 20% or 40% it would result in different decisions with respect to, say, culling of animals or implementation of a vaccination programme. In that case, a precision of 5% would be needed. Note that the logic described here does not involve testing a specific hypothesis.

The *confidence level* is usually set to 95% and it indicates how certain we want to be that the confidence interval calculated for the sample estimate includes the true value. It can be used for single parameters, such as prevalence, as well as for comparison between value estimates for different levels of a risk factor, such as a comparison of disease prevalence between two breeds of cats.

The *power* of a statistical test refers to how likely it is that a statistically significant difference of a given magnitude will be detected, under the assumption that it does indeed exist. A power of 80% is often used, which means that the study has an 80% chance of detecting a difference of at least as large a magnitude as the one assumed.

The *design effect* quantifies the effect of the sampling strategy on the variability in the data. As mentioned above, it is calculated as the ratio between the variance obtained using a particular sampling strategy and the variance one would have obtained through simple random sampling. It expresses the required change in sample size when using stratified or cluster sampling approaches. The basic principle in the case of cluster sampling is that the more similar animals are within a cluster and the larger the number of animals from each cluster, the higher will be the numeric value of the design effect. It is influenced by the sample size within clusters and the intracluster correlation coefficient which quantifies the homogeneity within clusters.

Sample size for determining population parameters

Estimation of level of disease occurrence

If the objective is to estimate proportions such as disease prevalence or incidence risk, the following information is required. First, a guesstimate of the
probable proportion of animals with the disease (P) has to be obtained which
can be used to calculate an estimate of the expected variation. If it is not
known, P = 0.5 can be used as this gives the largest sample size (see Table 7.2
above). Then, the level of desired precision L has to be decided. It is usually
specified as the number of percentage points around the expected estimate
(*absolute precision*) rather than as a percentage of the expected value (*relative
precision*). Finally, a decision has to be made as to the desired confidence level.
The choice is typically between 0.9, 0.95 and 0.99, with 0.95 usually being
used. If sampling strategies other than simple random sampling were used, a
design effect parameter should be used to adjust the sample size for sampling
design. In the case of stratified sampling, the variance typically has to be
adjusted downwards and with cluster or multistage sampling the variance has
to be adjusted upwards using the design effect as a multiplier of estimated
sample sizes.

Assuming an infinite population size, the formula for calculating the
required sample size n is presented in Equation 7.1. To be able to use it, the
parameters for variance [= $p(1-p)$] and precision (= L) have to be provided as
discussed above (note that both need to be scaled as proportions and not as
percentages). The value for Z reflects the desired confidence level, and values
of 1.65, 1.96 and 2.58 represent 90%, 95% and 99% confidence levels, respectively. If the sample size n is greater than 10% of the source population size,
use Equation 7.2 to obtain the sample size n'.

$$n = Z^2 \left[p(1-p)/L^2 \right] \tag{7.1}$$

where n is the sample size, Z is the Z-value reflecting the desired level of
confidence, L is the desired precision and p is the expected proportion.

$$n' = 1/[(1/n)+(1/N)] \tag{7.2}$$

where n' is the adjusted sample size, n is the sample size for an infinite population and N is the population size.

The following example demonstrates the use of the above equations. An
investigator has been asked to determine the proportion of cats in a population
associated with a veterinary practice that are serologically positive for infection with feline leukemia virus (FeLV). The desired absolute precision is ±5%
and the observed prevalence in similar cat populations has been reported to
be 10%. Applying Equation 7.1 indicates that about 138 cats will have to be
sampled to determine the proportion of FeLV positive cats in the veterinary
practice's cat population:

Table 7.3 Sample size for estimating level of disease occurrence at 95% confidence level assuming infinite population size

Expected prevalence (%)	Desired precision (%)		
	10	5	1
10	35	138	3457
20	61	246	6147
40	92	369	9220
60	92	369	9220
80	61	246	6147

If the total population at the practice is 500 cats, then a correction for finite populations needs to be applied, since the sample will involve more than 10% of the total population. From Equation 7.2, the corrected sample size is 108 animals.

$$n = 1.96^2 \times [0.1 \times (1 - 0.1)]/0.05^2 = 138$$

Although it is useful to understand the principles behind these calculations, the required sample sizes can also be obtained from tables or specialised epidemiological computer software such as OpenEpi (www.openepi.org) or WinEpiscope (www.clive.ed.ac.uk/winepiscope). Table 7.3 shows the sample sizes for different prevalence and absolute precision ranges at a 95% confidence level. As an example, to estimate the prevalence of disease in a large population to within ±5% at the 95% confidence level for an expected prevalence of 20%, it is necessary to examine a random sample of 246 animals.

The above calculations assume that the sensitivity and specificity of the disease diagnosis are both 100%. Jordan and McEwen (1998), Wagner and Salman (2004) and Humphry et al. (2004) discuss approaches for dealing with test uncertainty in sample size calculations.

Detecting disease in a population

During outbreak investigations or disease control/eradication programmes, or if testing the whole herd is too expensive, the objective is often to determine the presence or absence of disease. The basic concept is that if a particular disease is present in a population, it is usually possible to make assumptions about the likely minimum level of disease prevalence, based on experience from other infected populations or basic epidemiological principles. As an example, for a disease such as foot-and-mouth disease it is unlikely that less than 5% of animals will be infected in a herd that is kept as a single group and is not vaccinated (in fact the number is probably higher). Based on this assumption, a sample size can be calculated which has a certain likelihood to detect at least one of the infected animals in such a population. Equations 7.3 and 7.4 show the formulas for finite (<1000 animals) and infinite population sizes, respectively. Note that these formulas assume that diagnostic test specificity and sensitivity are both 100%. The case of less than 100% specificity is often not considered to be as much of a problem as lack of sensitivity, since any false positives would be identified during follow-up examination. Less than 100% sensitivity can be taken into account by using the sensitivity value to adjust the expected prevalence. As an example, if the sensitivity of the diagnostic test is 80%, only 80% of the prevalent cases will be detected, and therefore the sample size calculation needs to be tailored to a detectable prevalence value that is 0.8 of the expected prevalence.

$$n = \left(1 - \alpha^{1/D}\right)\left[N - \frac{1}{2}(D-1)\right] \qquad (7.3)$$

where n is the sample size, $\alpha = 1 -$ confidence level (as a proportion), N is the population size and D is the number of diseased animals (population size × minimum prevalence).

$$n = \ln\alpha/\ln(1-p) \qquad (7.4)$$

where n is the sample size, $\alpha = 1 -$ confidence level (as a proportion) and p is the expected minimum prevalence.

To simplify the process as mentioned above, computer programs or a table such as Table 7.4 can be used to perform these calculations. The interpretation of the sample size obtained from this table is that if no animal in the sample gives a positive test result, you can assume with 95% level of confidence that the disease is not present in the population.

Table 7.4 Sample size for estimating sample size for detecting presence of disease at 95% confidence level

Population size	Expected minimum prevalence (%)					
	0.1	1	2	5	10	20
10	10	10	10	10	10	8
50	50	50	48	35	22	12
100	100	96	78	45	25	13
500	500	225	129	56	28	14
1000	950	258	138	57	29	14
10000	2588	294	148	59	29	14
∞	2995	299	149	59	29	14

Maximum number of diseased animals in a population given all animals in the sample are negative

It may be relevant to determine how many diseased animals might be in a particular source population, despite all animals in a sample from that population having tested negative. The calculation shown in Equation 7.5 is similar to the method described above, as are the issues associated with less than 100% test sensitivity. It will allow an estimation of the maximum number of diseased animals D in a source population of size N at 95% confidence, given that all animals in a sample of size n are negative. Figure 7.2 shows how likely it is with relatively small sampling fractions of about 1–5% to misdiagnose an infected population as non-diseased.

$$D = \left[1 - (1-p)^{1/n}\right]\left[N - \frac{1}{2}(n-1)\right] \tag{7.5}$$

where n is the sample size, p is the expected prevalence, N is the population size and D is the number of diseased animals in the population.

Probability of not detecting disease

The disease status of a large population may be assessed through repeated testing of sample groups of animals. In this case, it would be useful to quantify

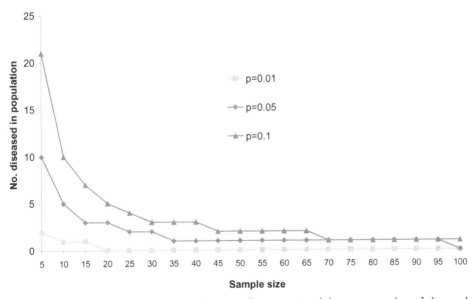

Figure 7.2 Relationship between sample size (all negative) and the upper number of diseased animals in the source population for different prevalence levels p (assuming 95% confidence level and a source population of $N = 1000$ animals).

Table 7.5 Probability of missing disease given different sample sizes from an infinite population

Expected prevalence (%)	Sample size					
	5	10	50	100	500	1000
1	0.95	0.90	0.61	0.37	0.01	0.00
2	0.90	0.82	0.36	0.13	0.00	
5	0.77	0.60	0.08	0.01		
10	0.59	0.35	0.01			
20	0.33	0.11	0.00			

the probability of failure to detect any positives in a series of samples from that population. The assumption in Equation 7.6 is that population size is infinite, and that data on the expected maximum prevalence p and sample size are available. Table 7.5 shows the resulting probability of failing to detect disease in a given sample for several combinations of expected prevalence and sample size. As an example, if one were to import multiple groups of 5 animals each from a population with 1% disease prevalence, 95% of the sample groups would not include any infected animals, and this could lead to the false conclusion that the source population is not infected.

$$\beta = (1 - p)^n \qquad (7.6)$$

where n is the sample size, p is the expected maximum prevalence and D is the number of diseased animals in the population.

Estimation of continuous-type population parameters

The calculation of the sample size for estimation of a continuous-type population parameter uses the same formula as for the estimation of level of disease occurrence, except that variance is calculated differently (see Equation 7.7). It is furthermore assumed that the parameter of interest is normally distributed.

$$n = Z^2 (\sigma/L^2) \qquad (7.7)$$

where n is the sample size, Z is the Z-value reflecting the desired level of confidence, σ is the standard deviation and L is the desired precision.

As an example, let us assume that an investigator would like to estimate average daily milk production in a dairy cow herd. The desired precision has been set to 1 kg, and a 95% confidence level will be used, meaning that $Z = 1.96$. The likely variance can be estimated using the approach described in the previous section. Assuming that the expectation is that about 95% of animals will be within 3 kg on either side of the average, this value represents about two standard deviations, so that one standard deviation becomes about 1.5 kg. Using the formula presented in Equation 7.7, the recommended sample size would be

$$n = 1.96^2 \times (1.5^2/0.5^2) = 8.6$$

in other words about 9 animals.

Sample size for effect estimation

Sample size calculations for estimation of effects can be based either on statistical hypothesis testing or estimation. The approaches described here use statistical hypothesis testing, and they therefore involve specification of statistical power. Estimation or precision-based approaches are presented in Dohoo *et al.* (2009).

Detecting a statistically significant difference between proportions

If the proportion of animals infected by a disease (= prevalence) is to be compared between two risk factor levels (exposed and non-exposed), the necessary sample size can be calculated using Equation 7.8. Data on the expected proportions are required, as well as a decision in relation to appropriate confidence level, typically 95% ($p \leq 0.05$) resulting in a Z_α of 1.96 for a *two-tailed test*. The value for Z_β will be −0.84, representing a statistical power of 80% for a *one-tailed test*.

$$n = \left[Z_\alpha \sqrt{(2pq)} - Z_\beta \sqrt{(p_1 q_1 + p_2 q_2)} \right]^2 / (p_1 - p_2)^2 \qquad (7.8)$$

where n is the sample size (per group), Z_α is the Z-value for confidence level, Z_β is the Z-value for statistical power, p is the proportion for pooled data, p_i is the estimated proportion in group i and $q_i = 1 - p_i$.

The magnitude of sample sizes required when you are intending to compare proportions can be surprisingly high. As an example, the effect of a treatment on conception probability at first service is to be tested in dairy cows using a two-tailed test. The latter implies, in contrast to a one-tailed test, that estimates for the treated group larger as well as smaller as those for the untreated group, are to be identified. In this example, the assumed proportion in animals without treatment is 0.4, the desired confidence level 95% ($p \leq 0.05$) and the statistical power 80%. Using Equation 7.8, a sample size of 1513 animals per group would be required to detect a difference of 0.05 in conception probability. If proportions of 0.1 and 0.15 had been compared with each other, only 684 animals would be required per group.

Detecting a statistically significant difference between continuous-scale variables

The objective of a study may be to assess the impact of a treatment on milk production in dairy cows. In this case, the data collected in the study can be used to generate two probability distributions, one describing variation in milk production in treated animals and the other in untreated animals. The question is now whether the distributions are different, and this is usually determined by comparing their mean values, taking account of any overlap between the two distributions. This process involves statistical hypothesis testing with the null hypothesis being that there is no difference in the mean values of the two groups. To use Equation 7.9, a confidence level needs to be decided; as mentioned above, this is typically 95% ($p \leq 0.05$) resulting in a Z_α of 1.96 for a two-tailed test. The value for Z_β will be -0.84, representing a statistical power of 80% for a one-tailed test. An estimate of the standard deviation of the parameter of interest, and also of the difference between the means of the two groups is required.

$$n = 2\left[(Z_\alpha - Z_\beta)^2 \, \sigma^2 \big/ (\mu_1 - \mu_2)^2\right] \tag{7.9}$$

where n is the sample size (per group), Z_α is the Z-value for confidence level, Z_β is the Z-value for statistical power, σ is the estimated standard deviation in the population and μ_i is the estimated mean for group i.

Taking account of clustering and multivariable analysis

Studies conducted in animal populations often involve measurement at the level of the unit of interest such as an individual cow or some aggregate of these animals, such as a herd. The issue here is that the animals within these aggregates are likely to be more similar to each other with respect to these measurements than to animals from other aggregates. This also means that the number of aggregates (e.g. herds) chosen may be more influential than the number of animals within each aggregate (see discussion for cluster sampling). Standard sample size calculation methods assume independence of all sample units from each other, and would therefore underestimate the required sample size when using cluster sampling. As discussed earlier, the design effect expresses the relationship between the variance in such a study involving cluster sampling and what it would have been under simple random sampling. An adjusted sample size can be calculated using the formula from Dohoo *et al.* (2009) shown in Equation 7.10, which requires information on the dependence within aggregates quantified using the intracluster (or intraclass) correlation coefficient and the average sample size within clusters.

$$n' = n[1 + p(m - 1)] \tag{7.10}$$

where n' is the sample size adjusted for clustering, n is the original sample size assuming simple random sampling, ρ is the intracluster or intraclass correlation coefficient and m is the average number of animals per aggregate (e.g. herd).

Note that Equation 7.10 assumes that the risk factors are clustered at the aggregate level (e.g. dairy versus beef operation), which would in effect represent a high degree of clustering. But there may also be animal-level factors that are clustered, e.g. some farms may have a higher proportion of a particular breed than others. In this case, there is likely to be a lower degree of clustering, and the sample size adjustment described in Equation 7.10 may be too extreme. The investigator will then have to use their judgement with respect to the required amount of sample size adjustment, although if in doubt they could opt for the conservative estimate obtained from Equation 7.10.

Epidemiological studies are usually aimed at investigating multifactorial cause–effect relationships. As a consequence, they will be affected to a varying extent by the presence of confounding bias and potentially by interaction relationships in the data. This will also require an increase in sample size, and Dohoo *et al.* (2009) recommend an increase by 15% for moderately strong confounders that have an odds ratio of between 0.5 and 2 with outcome and the exposure. Further calculations can be found in Dohoo *et al.* (2009).

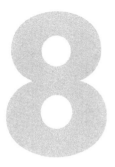

Interpreting diagnostic tests

Learning objectives

After completing this chapter, you will be able to:

- Define and differentiate the concepts of sensitivity and specificity.
- Calculate predictive value and explain how predictive value is determined by sensitivity, specificity and the prevalence of the condition being evaluated.
- Understand the concept of likelihood ratios.
- Interpret ROC curves.
- Understand the use and implications of multiple testing.

Introduction

The ability to diagnose disease is one of the most important decision support tools that a veterinarian has available. The outcome of the diagnostic process is a diagnosis indicating whether an animal is considered normal or not normal. This could relate not only to disease or infection status but also to production performance or quality of life from an animal welfare perspective, but in this chapter we will assume for simplicity that the diagnosis relates to a disease.

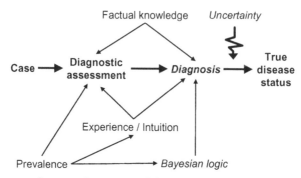

Figure 8.1   Factors influencing the process of diagnostic reasoning.

A diagnosis is almost always associated with some degree of uncertainty, and therefore the diagnostic outcome has to be the probability that the animal has a particular disease. The diagnosis will inform a decision which may be about whether to treat or to do nothing, to evaluate further, to wait or in some cases whether to euthanase. The tools the veterinarian uses in addition to the diagnostic assessment to come to a diagnosis include factual knowledge, experience and intuition (see Figure 8.1). Although most of these tools do not lend themselves to quantitative analysis, all diagnostic tests will have quantitative diagnostic performance characteristics and these can be combined using Bayesian logic with disease probabilities, such as population prevalence, to calculate disease probability. It is the aim of the diagnostician to combine the diagnostic tools so that the probability of a correct diagnosis is maximised, i.e. the uncertainty associated with the diagnosis is minimised. The diagnostic assessment includes history taking, physical examination and diagnostic imaging as well as any diagnostic tests performed in the laboratory. The principles discussed in this chapter apply to any of the findings derived from the diagnostic assessment, not only to laboratory tests.

Diagnostic tests

A diagnostic test is a more or less objective method for reducing diagnostic uncertainty, and includes all tools that are used during the diagnostic assessment. As the consequential decision is typically dichotomous (e.g. to treat or not), the outcome of the diagnostic process often is also interpreted as a dichotomous variable, i.e. that the animal has a particular disease or not. The unit of measurement of the diagnostic tool itself may already be dichotomous, such as presence or absence of bacteria, thereby considerably facilitating interpretation. Many diagnostic tests use biological markers, such as serum anti-

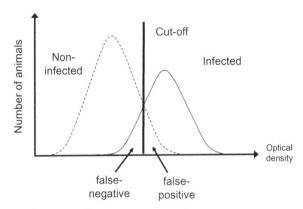

Figure 8.2 Test result measured on a continuous scale.

body levels or blood biochemistry, and more recently molecular and genetic methods as well. If the diagnostic tool generates continuous-scale measures, such as serum antibody levels or somatic cell counts, a cut-off value has to be determined so that the result can be interpreted on a dichotomous scale. For a continuous-scale clinical measurement, any cut-off point is likely to result in overlap between healthy and diseased animals (see Figure 8.2). The consequences of this situation are that uncertainty in addition to any other potential sources of measurement error (such as operator error) is being introduced. It is desirable to quantify this relationship between diagnostic test result and 'true' disease status so that the clinician can take account of this uncertainty when interpreting test results.

The performance of a diagnostic method is often summarised using the following three terms. The *accuracy* refers to the closeness between test result and 'true' clinical state. The *misclassification bias* is a measure of the systematic deviation from 'true' disease status. The *precision* or *repeatability* represents the degree of fluctuation of the results obtained through repeated testing of the same biological sample. Such variability may be the result of poor adherence to test protocols within or between laboratories. Any evaluation of diagnostic tests needs a measure of the 'true' condition of animals, which is usually called the *gold standard* or *reference test*. But is important to realise that most of the time it is impossible to define with 100% accuracy what the true diagnosis should be. In addition, there may also be disagreement among experts, e.g. in the case of mastitis where the presence of a particular pathogen or the presence of an inflammatory response in the udder could be defined as the gold standard. Table 8.1 shows the structure and notation for the 2 × 2 table which will be used in this chapter for analyses related to diagnostic test evaluation and interpretation.

Table 8.1   Presentation of data as 2 × 2 table for evaluation of diagnostic tests

Disease status	Diagnostic test result		Total
	Positive	**Negative**	
Disease	a	b	m_1
No disease	c	d	m_0
Total	n_1	n_0	n

Evaluating diagnostic tests

To assess a diagnostic test or compare a number of different tests, it is necessary to apply the tests as well as the gold standard or reference test to a sample of animals from a population with a typical disease spectrum. The diagnostician should be aware that the results of such evaluations can differ between populations, as a result of differences in severity or stage of disease at the population level. This is of particular relevance when evaluations were conducted under experimental conditions. It is also important to recognise that such comparisons assume that the gold standard is a more accurate test than the tests that are included in the evaluation. This means that a test which in reality is accurate might appear to perform poorly if evaluated using an imperfect gold standard. In such situations, it may be preferable to compare different methods without one of them being interpreted as the gold standard. Instead, one would assess the agreement between both diagnostic methods. The methods described here only apply to qualitative outcomes, i.e. test positive or negative, and diseased or non-diseased. Methods for assessing agreement between diagnostic methods measured on a quantitative scale are described in Nielsen *et al.* (2004) and Dohoo *et al.* (2009).

Studies for evaluating diagnostic tests use different approaches for selecting diseased and non-diseased animals, which impact on the validity of inferences in relation to test performance. The options include applying both the gold standard and the test to be evaluated to all animals selected from a population, or to apply the gold standard test only to a sample of test positive and negative animals. Dohoo *et al.* (2009) and Kraemer (1992) provide detailed discussions of the various approaches.

Comparison with a gold standard

The characteristics of the evaluated test relative to the gold standard test are quantified through sensitivity and specificity. *Sensitivity* (*Se*) relates to animals that have the disease, and among these it expresses the proportion of animals that have a positive test (see Equation 8.1). In other words, it is the ability of the evaluated test to correctly identify diseased animals and therefore gives an indication of how many false-negative results can be expected.

$$Se = a/m_1 \qquad (8.1)$$

where Se is test sensitivity, a is the number of animals that are test positive and diseased (see Table 8.1) and m_1 is the number animals that are diseased (see Table 8.1). Note that this evaluation is about diagnostic and not analytic sensitivity. The latter concept is used in laboratory situations to express the ability of a test to detect low concentrations of chemical compounds.

Specificity (Sp), on the other hand, relates to animals without the disease, and among these it expresses the proportion of animals which test negative (see Equation 8.2). It represents the ability of a diagnostic test to correctly identify non-diseased animals and gives an indication of how many false positive results can be expected.

$$Sp = d/m_0 \qquad (8.2)$$

where Sp is test specificity, d is the number of animals that are test negative and are not diseased (see Table 8.1) and m_0 is the number of animals that are not diseased (see Table 8.1). Diagnostic specificity differs from analytic specificity, in that the latter refers to the ability of laboratory tests to distinguish between different compounds.

Diagnostic sensitivity (Se) and specificity (Sp) are inversely related and in the case of test results measured on a continuous scale they can be influenced by changing the cut-off value. An increase in sensitivity will usually result in a decrease in specificity, and vice versa. The optimum cut-off value depends on the diagnostic strategy. If the primary objective is to find diseased animals, meaning that false negatives are to be minimised (i.e. rule out disease) and a limited number of false positives is acceptable, a test with a high sensitivity and good specificity is required. A test with high sensitivity will allow the diagnostician to have high confidence in a negative result. But a positive result will not be as reliable, and any positives may therefore have to be examined by other diagnostic tests. For example, diagnostic tests for rabies should have a high sensitivity, since consequences of false-negative results can be very serious. In contrast, if the objective is to make sure that every test positive is 'truly' diseased (= rule in disease), the diagnostic test should have a high specificity and good sensitivity, meaning false positives are to be minimised whereas a limited number of false negatives may be acceptable. Such tests should be used if false-positive results have important consequences, e.g. of an economic or welfare nature, for the animal or its owner. As an example,

Table 8.2   Presentation of data for analysis of agreement between two diagnostic tests

Test 1	Test 2		Total
	Positive	Negative	
Positive	a	b	$a + b$
Negative	c	d	$c + d$
Total	$a + c$	$b + d$	n

farmers will not be allowed to sell their cattle for a period as soon as at least one of their animals has shown a positive tuberculin test reaction. If it then turns out that these animals were false positives, a farmer may have incurred economic losses because of the inability to trade cattle.

Agreement

It frequently happens in diagnostic test evaluation that no acceptable gold standard is available, and it may therefore become necessary to evaluate agreement between the tests, e.g. with one of the tests being a generally accepted diagnostic method. The kappa (κ) test is a statistical method for assessing the agreement between diagnostic methods measured on a dichotomous scale. It measures the proportion of agreement beyond that to be expected by chance. The statistic ranges from 0 to 1 with a κ value of about 0.4–0.6 indicating moderate agreement. Higher κ values are interpreted as good agreement and lower values as poor agreement. The κ test can also be used e.g. to evaluate agreement between clinical diagnoses based on radiographic images made by the same clinician on repeated examination of the same image or between different clinicians. Table 8.2 shows how the data should be presented for an analysis of agreement between two diagnostic tests.

The calculation of the κ statistic (see Equation 8.5) requires calculation of the observed proportion of agreement (see Equation 8.3) and the expected proportion (see Equation 8.4) assuming chance agreement.

$$OP = (a + d)/n \tag{8.3}$$

where OP is the observed proportion of agreement, a is the number of occasions both tests are positive, d is the number of occasions both tests are negative and n is the total number of samples (see Table 8.2).

$$EP = \{[(a + b)(a + c)]/n + [(c + d)(b + d)]/n\}/n \tag{8.4}$$

Table 8.3 Data for analysis of agreement between two ELISA tests for diagnosis of *Neospora caninum* infection in cattle

		ELISA A	
		positive	**negative**
ELISA B	positive	41	9
	negative	69	187

where EP is the expected proportion of agreement, *a* is the number of occasions both tests are positive, *b* is the number of occasions test 1 is negative and test 2 is positive, *c* is the number of occasions test 1 is positive and test 2 is negative, *d* is the number of occasions both tests are negative and *n* is the total number of samples (see Table 8.2).

$$\kappa = (OP - EP)/(1 - EP) \tag{8.5}$$

where κ is the kappa statistic, OP is the observed proportion of agreement (see Equation 8.3) and EP is the expected proportion of agreement (see Equation 8.4).

The following example calculation for the κ statistic is derived from data in Reichel and Pfeiffer (2002) based on the comparison of two ELISA tests for diagnosis of *Neospora caninum* infection in cattle (see Table 8.3).

$$OP = (41 + 187)/306 = 0.75$$

$$EP = \{[(41 + 9) \times (41 + 69)]/306 + [(69 + 187) \times (9 + 187)]/306\}/306 = 0.59$$

$$\kappa = (0.75 - 0.59)/(1 - 0.59) = 0.37$$

The calculations presented above yield a value of 0.37 for κ, indicating poor agreement between both tests. Note that this analysis will not allow inferences in relation to false classification, as neither of the two methods represents a gold standard. ELISA A seems to diagnose a lot more positives than ELISA B.

Test performance and interpretation at the individual animal level

Predictive values can be used to take account of test characteristics during the diagnostic decision process. They quantify the probability that a test result for a particular animal correctly identifies the condition or disease of interest. The predictive value of a positive test result (PV⁺) expresses the proportion of test-positive animals which really have the disease (see Equation 8.6). Given availability of data on true prevalence, test sensitivity and specificity values, PV⁺ can be calculated based on Bayes' theorem of conditional probabilities as described in Equation 8.7.

$$PV^+ = a/n_1 \qquad (8.6)$$

where PV⁺ is the predictive value of a positive test, a is the number of animals that are test-positive and diseased, and n_1 is the number of animals that are test-positive (see Table 8.1).

$$PV^+ = (Prev_{true} \times Se)/[(Prev_{true} \times Se) + (1 - Prev_{true})(1 - Sp)] \qquad (8.7)$$

where PV⁺ is the predictive value of a positive test, $Prev_{true}$ is the true disease prevalence, Se is the test sensitivity and Sp is the test specificity.

The predictive value of a negative test result (PV⁻) represents the proportion of test-negative animals that do not have the disease (see Equation 8.8). If the sensitivity and specificity of the test and the true prevalence are known, the negative predictive value can be calculated using Equation 8.9.

$$PV^- = d/n_0 \qquad (8.8)$$

where PV^- is the predictive value of a negative test, d is the number of animals that are test-negative and not diseased and n_0 is the number of animals that are test-negative (see Table 8.1).

$$PV^- = (1 - Prev_{true} \times Sp)/[(1 - Prev_{true} \times Sp) + Prev_{true}(1 - Se)] \qquad (8.9)$$

where PV^- is the predictive value of a negative test, $Prev_{true}$ is the true disease prevalence, Se is the test sensitivity and Sp is the test specificity.

It is important to remember that predictive values are used for interpretation at the individual animal level and cannot be used to compare tests, since they depend on prevalence, as well as on sensitivity and specificity. In fact, prevalence is probably more important in practical terms because it is likely to vary substantially between populations, whereas sensitivity and specificity will do so much less, if at all. The combination of the various probabilities is difficult to perform intuitively, which is why the importance of prevalence is often ignored when interpreting test results, and instead the intuitive focus is placed only on test sensitivity or specificity. In fact, the consequence of this conditional probability relationship is that one could argue that in the presence of low prevalence situations any positive test result needs to be interpreted very

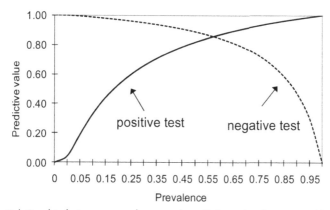

Figure 8.3 Relationship between prevalence and predictive value for a test with 90% sensitivity and 80% specificity.

carefully, as it will have a low positive predictive value. The reason for this effect is that there are many more animals without than with the disease in the population, and therefore the false positives generated by less than 100% specificity are likely to represent a larger proportion of the total test positives than the true positives.

In the following example the test is assumed to have 95% sensitivity and 90% specificity, which is not an unusual set of test characteristics. Applying this test in a population with 30% disease prevalence will result in a predictive value for a positive test of 80% and of 98% for a negative test. If disease prevalence is only 3%, and test characteristics remain the same, the predictive value of a positive test will be 23% and for a negative test 99.8%. The key issue here is the 90% specificity, which will produce 10% false positives among those that do not have the disease. Therefore, the higher the proportion of animals without the disease (i.e. low prevalence), the higher will be the proportion of false positives among animals testing positive. For a test with 90% sensitivity and 80% specificity, Figure 8.3 shows that the positive predictive value remains below 40% for prevalence levels up to 15%. On the other hand, the negative predictive value for the same test only drops below 95% once prevalence increases above 30%.

Prevalence estimation and diagnostic tests

True prevalence is the proportion of animals within a population that have the disease. In reality, this information is impossible to obtain, since the assessment of disease status requires the use of a diagnostic method. Instead, as a consequence of tests producing false negatives and false positives, only the proportion of animals in the population that give a positive test result can be calculated, which is called the *apparent prevalence*. Its value may be higher or lower than the true prevalence, or equal to it. Estimates of the true prevalence can be obtained by adjusting the apparent prevalence through taking account of test sensitivity and specificity as shown in Equation 8.10.

$$\text{Prev}_{\text{true}} = [\text{Prev}_{\text{apparent}} + (Sp - 1)]/[Sp + (Se - 1)] \tag{8.10}$$

where $\text{Prev}_{\text{true}}$ = true disease prevalence, $\text{Prev}_{\text{apparent}}$ = apparent disease prevalence, Se = test sensitivity and Sp = test specificity.

In clinical epidemiology, the terms prior prevalence, prior probability, pre-test prevalence or pre-test probability are used instead of true prevalence to refer to the probability that an animal has the disease before a test has been used. Once a test has been applied, the post-test prevalence, post-test probability or posterior probability can be calculated (= apparent prevalence).

Clinical perspective on interpretation of diagnostic tests

When interpreting a diagnostic test, the clinician needs to recognise the importance of prevalence or *prior probability* of disease, in addition to sensitivity and specificity. As discussed above, if the prior probability is extremely small, a positive test result is not very meaningful and must be followed up by a highly *specific* test. It is therefore important that the prior probability before testing is increased as much as possible, by taking into account specific population disease risk characteristics as well as clinical findings. The following sequence of steps describes how probabilities can be incorporated into diagnostic decision-making (Gross 1999). The basic principle is that the outcome of the process is a diagnosis expressed as a probability of the animal having a particular disease which in turn will inform a particular action that is to be taken. If possible, the clinician should define *a priori* the probability threshold values for different action plans. Figure 8.4 shows the probability of disease

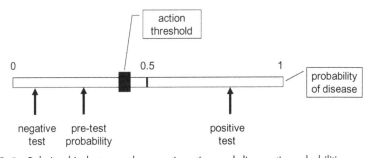

Figure 8.4 Relationship between therapeutic action and diagnostic probabilities.

(i.e. the outcome of the diagnostic process) as a horizontal bar representing the range of possible probability values from 0 to 1. In this hypothetical example, it was decided on economic and welfare grounds to implement a parasite treatment if the probability of disease was at least 40%, and to do nothing if it was below that value. The purpose of the diagnostic test is now to determine whether for this animal the probability of disease is above or below the action threshold. To do this the first parameter to consider is the *pre-test probability*. This parameter basically indicates how likely it is that the animal has the disease, based on the information that is available so far. The pre-test probability is the result of combining various probabilities, the first of which is usually the prevalence of the particular disease in the population. That probability is then revised by taking into account various other factors known to influence the likelihood of disease. These may be e.g. specific risk factors such as breed or age of the animal, or the findings from the clinical examination. The skill of the clinician is to combine these findings such that a meaningful pre-test probability can be produced. If the pre-test probability is already above the action threshold, it may not be necessary to apply the test. If that is not the case (as in the current example), the pre-test probability, test sensitivity and specificity should be combined to calculate positive and negative predictive values for the two possible test outcomes before applying the test. Should these remain on the left side of the action threshold in Figure 8.4, there is no rationale for using the diagnostic test. In the current example, a positive result represents an 80% probability that the animal has the disease and would therefore be beyond the action threshold, thereby justifying the application of the test. So, if the test is positive, the animal would be vaccinated.

Methods for choosing cut-off values

The criteria for deriving cut-off values from diagnostic tools measuring quantities on a continuous scale such as optical densities of ELISA tests can be based on a range of different methods. The most commonly applied technique used to be the Gaussian distribution method. This has now largely been replaced by the diagnostic or predictive value method which uses the receiver-operating characteristic (ROC) curve. Figure 8.5 shows an example of data for an ELISA test for diagnosis of *Neospora caninum* infection (Reichel and Pfeiffer 2002). It demonstrates the extensive overlap between the distribution of test values for gold standard positive and negative animals. In this case, a cut-off of 0.15 maximises sensitivity and specificity. Note that the gold standard is another test which itself is not 100% accurate.

The Gaussian distribution method can be used to derive a cut-off value using only test results from a disease-free population. It involves first

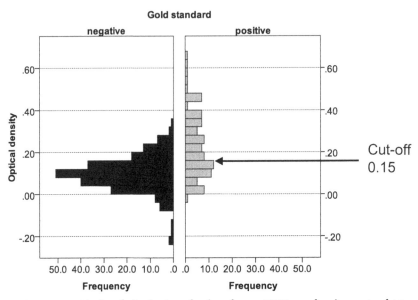

Figure 8.5 Pyramid plot of distribution of values for an ELISA test for diagnosis of *Neospora caninum* infection in cattle.

producing a histogram to confirm the Gaussian shape of the data and then computing the mean and standard deviation of the test results. The upper and lower limits of the test results are defined using two standard deviations from the mean. That means 95% of values in the disease-free population will have values within this interval. The other values would be classified as abnormal. The advantage of the Gaussian distribution method is that only data from a known disease-free population are required. Its disadvantages include that it predefines the specificity at a fixed value such as 97.5% in this example while ignoring sensitivity, and that it may misrepresent non-normally distributed test value data.

The diagnostic or predictive value method is considered the most clinically sound approach. With this technique, the cut-off is selected so that it produces a sensitivity and specificity which is optimal for a particular diagnostic strategy. This can be done using the information contained in a ROC curve. The choice of a suitable cut-off will be influenced by whether false positives or negatives are considered less desirable by the clinician. The advantages of the predictive value method include that it can be applied regardless of the statistical distributional characteristics of the test values. It uses realistic, clinical data for the development of the cut-off values, and includes information on the diseased as well as the non-diseased population. Most importantly, it allows a clinician to select a cut-off which suits particular diagnostic objectives. The disadvantage of the method is that it requires a clinician to have a good understanding of this method to be able to choose between different cut-offs.

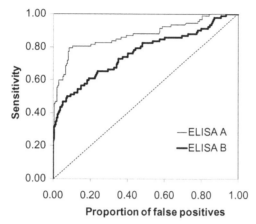

Figure 8.6 Receiver-operating characteristic (ROC) curves for two ELISA tests. Reprinted from Reichel and Pfeiffer (2002), copyright 2002, with permission from Elsevier.

The ROC curve mentioned in the context of the predictive value method consists of an *x-y* plot of sensitivity and proportion false positive (1 – specificity) value pairs for different cut-off values (see Figure 8.6). The calculations necessary to obtain these value pairs require data on test values and true disease status for a sufficiently large number of animals. For each possible cut-off value, animals' individual test values are then interpreted as test positive or negative, and used to calculate sensitivity/false-positive proportion values for the corresponding cut-off. This produces a list of sensitivity/false-positive proportion value pairs, each representing another cut-off. These value pairs are then plotted as points on an *x-y* plot with proportion false positives on the x-axis and sensitivity on the y-axis. A ROC curve is then produced by drawing a line connecting the points in sequential order of change in cut-off value. Since the respective cut-off values are usually not shown on the ROC plot, it is important to keep in mind that there is a particular cut-off value behind each of the points on the curve. A perfect diagnostic test should have 100% sensitivity and 0% false positives, and therefore reach the upper left corner of the *x-y* plot. A diagonal ROC curve (from lower left to upper right corner) indicates a diagnostic test which does not produce any useful differentiation between diseased and non-diseased animals. The area under the ROC curve can be used to quantify overall test accuracy. The larger this area, the better is the test. The ROC curve allows identification of cut-off values appropriate for different diagnostic strategies. If false negatives and positives are equally undesirable, a cut-off associated with a point on the ROC curve which is closest to the upper left corner of the *x-y* chart should be selected. Assuming that false positives are more undesirable, a cut-off associated with a point further to the left on the ROC curve should be used. If false negatives are more undesirable, the cut-off should be set to a value associated with a point towards the right on the ROC curve. Different diagnostic tests can be compared by plotting their ROC curves. The diagnostic test whose ROC curve comes closest to the upper left corner and which therefore has the largest area under the curve is usually the best test. In the example presented in Figure 8.6, ELISA A differentiates better between infected and non-infected animals than ELISA B. A more detailed discussion of ROC analysis is presented in Greiner *et al.* (2000).

Likelihood ratios

The purpose of a diagnostic test is to influence the clinician's opinion about whether or not the animal has the disease. This means that it is used to modify the opinion the clinician had before obtaining the test result in relation to the probability of the animal having the disease, i.e. it is a modifier of the *pre-test probability*, as described earlier. For this purpose, presenting the test result as positive or negative will not be that useful, because the result could still be a false positive or negative. What is needed is a quantity that gives the clinician an idea how likely it is that the test result could be obtained from a diseased animal compared with a non-diseased animal. This is expressed by the *likelihood ratio* (LR) which can be calculated for negative as well as positive test results, and also for ordinal- or continuous-scale test values. Assuming positive/negative test outcomes, the likelihood ratio for a positive test result (LR$^+$) is calculated by dividing the probability of a positive test result in animals with the disease (= sensitivity) by the probability of the test result among animals without the disease (= 1 – specificity) (see Equation 8.11). The result is interpreted as how likely it is to find a positive test result in diseased compared with non-diseased individuals. The likelihood ratio of a negative test result (LR$^-$) is calculated as the ratio between (1 – sensitivity) and specificity (see Equation 8.12). This result is then interpreted as how likely it is to find a negative test result in diseased compared with non-diseased animals. LR$^-$ is used less frequently than LR$^+$. The LR does not depend on prevalence, and provides a quantitative measure of the diagnostic information contained in a particular test result by combining diagnostic sensitivity and specificity into a single value.

$$LR^+ = Se/(1 - Sp) \tag{8.11}$$

where LR^+ is the likelihood ratio for a positive test result, Se is the test sensitivity and Sp is the test specificity.

$$LR^- = (1 - Se)/Sp \tag{8.12}$$

where LR^- is the likelihood ratio for a negative test result, Se is the test sensitivity and Sp is the test specificity.

Likelihood ratios can be calculated using single cut-off values, so that one obtains only one pair of likelihood ratios for a particular diagnostic test, one for a positive test result (LR^+) and another for a negative test result (LR^-). More powerful information can be extracted from the diagnostic test by using multilevel likelihood ratios. In this case every test value, or more often several sequential ranges of test values, will have its own LR^+ and LR^- values. The main advantage of the multilevel likelihood ratio method is that it allows the clinician to take account of the degree of abnormality, rather than just use crude categories such as test-positive or -negative. It is then possible when estimating the probability of disease presence (i.e. post-test probability) to place more emphasis on extremely high or low rather than on borderline test values. For example, an LR^+ value around 1 will not allow meaningful differentiation between diseased and non-diseased animals. Such LR values are often associated with test values around the cut-off point which with the traditional positive/negative interpretation of a diagnostic test would have been attributed to one of the two possible test categories. In contrast, an LR of 10 will provide strong indication of disease presence and would typically be obtained for test values further away from the aforementioned cut-off value. The multilevel likelihood ratio values can be calculated in a category-specific or cumulative fashion. Category-specific values are calculated as the ratio between the proportion of diseased animals and the proportion of non-diseased animals within each category's particular range of test values. If the cumulative method is used, sensitivity and specificity values are recalculated for different cut-offs and then Equations 8.11 and 8.12 are applied for each.

If used in combination with the initial expectation of the probability that an animal has a certain condition (= pre-test probability), a revised estimate of the probability of the condition (= post-test probability) can be calculated. In order to perform the revision of the pre-test probability, it first has to be converted into pre-test odds as described in Equation 8.13. The result is then multiplied with the likelihood ratio associated with a particular test value to produce an estimate of the post-test odds. This in turn then has to be converted back into a probability as shown in Equation 8.14.

$$\text{Odds} = \text{Probability}(1 - \text{Probability}) \tag{8.13}$$

$$\text{Probability} = \text{Odds}/(1 + \text{Odds}) \tag{8.14}$$

As an example, an ELISA test can be used for detection of *Neospora caninum* infection in cattle, a significant cause of abortion. A particular dairy farmer is known to have a *Neospora* prevalence of about 5% in the cow herd.

A blood sample from a cow that is to be sold produces an ELISA optical density (OD) value of 0.28. The probability that the cow is indeed infected with *Neospora caninum* can be calculated using the standard cut-off of 0.15 for this test or using the category-specific likelihood ratio for the actual test result. Based on the first method, assuming a cut-off of OD = 0.15 the test result is interpreted as positive. Given a known test sensitivity of 64% and specificity of 76% a positive predictive value of 12% can be calculated using Equation 8.7 as shown below. Note that it is also possible to convert the sensitivity and specificity values into a single cut-off value LR^+, and the PV^+ can then be calculated as described below.

$$PV^+ = (0.05 \times 0.64)/[(0.05 \times 0.64) + (1 - 005) \times (1 - 0.76)] = 0.12$$

To use a likelihood ratio approach, the known *Neospora* prevalence in this herd needs to be converted into pre-test odds as shown in Equation 8.13:

$$\text{Pre-test odds} = 0.05/(1 - 0.05) = 0.05$$

Next, a likelihood ratio value for a positive test has to be obtained for the test result of OD = 0.28 from Table 8.4.

The pre-test odds and the LR^+ value have to be multiplied to give the post-test odds, as follows:

$$\text{Post-test odds} = 0.05 \times 3.5 = 0.18$$

For ease of interpretation, the post-test odds is now converted back into a post-test probability as in Equation 8.14:

$$\text{Post-test probability} = 0.18/(1 + 0.18) = 0.15$$

The result of this calculation is now that the animal has a 15% chance of being infected, a value that is slightly higher than was obtained on the basis

Table 8.4 Likelihood ratio values for a positive test for optical density value ranges for a *Neospora caninum* ELISA test

	Optical density value ranges						
	< = 0.1	0.1–0.16	0.16–0.2	0.2–0.24	0.24–0.27	0.27–0.3	>0.3
LR⁺	0.37	0.75	1	1.5	2.8	3.5	65

of the single cut-off. In this case due to the low prevalence, the application of the likelihood ratio method does not greatly improve confidence in the test interpretation. It could be argued, though, that this relatively small difference is also a reflection of the poor overall performance of this particular test.

The calculation of post-test probabilities can be greatly facilitated by using a nomogram as shown in Figure 8.7. In the example shown, a test result was expressed as a likelihood ratio value for a positive test result of 10. The pre-test or prior probability as a result of knowledge of the population prevalence or clinical examination was assumed to be 20%. The post-test probability is obtained by drawing a straight line from the pre-test probability via the LR^+ value through to the resulting post-test probability of 75%.

The relationship between pre-test probability and various LR^+ values is summarised in Table 8.5. It demonstrates that with a low pre-test probability such as 5%, it is difficult even with a fairly high LR^+ of 10 to reach a high probability for diagnosing an animal as diseased. In fact, given a likelihood ratio for a positive test of 3, one would need at least a 30% pre-test probability to be more than 50% confident that an animal has the disease.

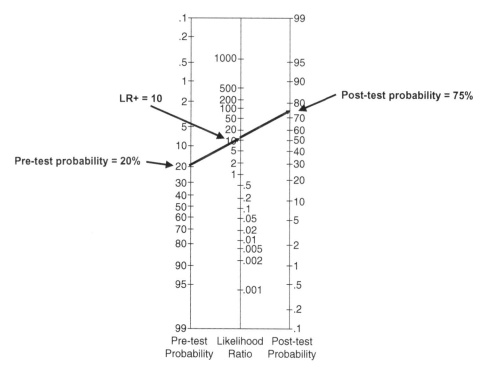

Figure 8.7 Nomogram for post-test probability calculation using likelihood ratios of a positive test result.

Table 8.5   Post-test probabilities for different pre-test probability and likelihood ratio for a positive test value combinations

		Pre-test probability (%)					
		5	**10**	**20**	**30**	**50**	**70**
Likelihood ratio for a positive test	**10**	34	53	71	81	91	96
	3	14	25	43	56	75	88
	1	5	10	20	30	50	70
	0.3	1.5	3.2	7	11	23	41
	0.1	0.5	1	2.5	4	9	19

Combining diagnostic test results

Different diagnostic methods can be used in combination to allow improved diagnosis through strategic decisions about interpretation of the results. These approaches include using different tests for the same disease problem in a single animal, using different tests each identifying different disease problems in a single animal or using the same test for a specific disease problem applied to several animals or the same animal over time.

Different tests for the same disease problem in a single animal

In the same animal, different diagnostic methods for the same disease are frequently used in combination to increase the clinician's confidence in a specific diagnosis for that animal. If this is done in a qualitative manner, it is very difficult to take full advantage of the combined information. Parallel and series interpretation can be used to combine the information provided by the individual test results. In this context it is essential to recognise that these methods relate to usage of different tests for the same disease at the same time in a single animal. The tests should be independent of each other and should therefore measure different biological parameters associated with the same disease, e.g. one may be an ELISA test for tuberculosis measuring serum antibodies and the other the tuberculin skin test measuring cell-mediated immunity.

Parallel and series interpretation

With parallel test interpretation, an animal is considered to have the disease if one or more tests are positive. This means the animal is being asked to 'prove' that it is healthy. The technique is recommended for rapid assessment, because the animal is considered positive after the first test that produces a positive result. If the first test is negative, the second test is still necessary. Parallel test interpretation will increase sensitivity and the predictive value of a negative test result, so that disease is less likely to be missed. But on the other hand it does reduce specificity and the predictive value of a positive test, hence false-positive diagnoses will be more likely. As a consequence, if enough tests are conducted, an apparent abnormality can be found in virtually every animal even if it is completely 'normal'. The combined test sensitivity/specificity values for two tests can be calculated as shown in Equations 8.15 and 8.16, based on Nielsen *et al.* (2004).

$$Se_{par} = 1 - (1 - Se_x) \times (1 - Se_y) \qquad (8.15)$$

$$Sp_{par} = Sp_x \times Sp_y \qquad (8.16)$$

where Se_{par} is the combined sensitivity based on parallel interpretation, Sp_{par} is the combined specificity based on parallel interpretation, Se_{xy} is the sensitivity of test x or y and Sp_{xy} is the specificity of test x or y.

With serial test interpretation, the animal is considered to have the disease if all tests are positive. In other words, the animal is being asked to 'prove' that it has the condition. Series testing can be used if no rapid assessment is necessary, because for an animal to be classified as positive all test results have to be obtained. If some of the tests are expensive or risky, testing can be stopped as soon as one test is negative. This method maximises specificity and positive predictive value, which means that more confidence can be attributed to positive results. It reduces sensitivity and negative predictive value, and it therefore becomes more likely that diseased animals are being missed. Likelihood ratios can be applied to the interpretation of serial testing by using the post-test odds resulting from a particular test as the pre-test odds for the next test in the series. The combined test sensitivity/specificity values for two tests can be calculated as shown in Equations 8.17 and 8.18, based on Nielsen *et al.* (2004).

$$Se_{ser} = Se_x \times Se_y \qquad (8.17)$$

$$Sp_{ser} = 1 - (1 - Sp_x) \times (1 - Sp_y) \qquad (8.18)$$

where Se_{ser} is the combined sensitivity based on serial interpretation, Sp_{ser} is the combined specificity based on serial interpretation, Se_{xy} is the sensitivity of test x or y, and Sp_{xy} is the specificity of test x or y.

The effects of interpreting each test on its own, in parallel or in series on the predictive values of two independent diagnostic tests for the same disease are compared in Table 8.6. In this example, a disease prevalence of 20% is assumed. Test A has a moderate sensitivity of 80% and a poor specificity of 60%, resulting in a very poor positive predictive value if the test is used alone. Test B has good sensitivity (90%) and specificity (90%), producing a better but still less than desirable positive predictive value. A parallel interpretation

Table 8.6   Example of parallel and series interpretation of a diagnostic test

Test	Sensitivity (%)	Specificity (%)	Positive predictive value (%)*	Negative predictive value (%)*
A	80	60	33	92
B	90	90	69	97
Parallel	98	54	35	99
Series	72	96	82	93

*Assuming 20% prevalence.

of the two test results improves the predictive value of negative tests from 92% for test A and 97% for test B to a combined level of 99%. This means any test-negatives almost certainly will not have the disease. But the positive predictive value is still only 35%, which means that parallel test interpretation positives should be evaluated carefully. A series interpretation of the results of both tests substantially improves the predictive value of a test-positive to 82%, so that it becomes useful from a diagnostic perspective. It results in a slight drop in the negative predictive value. Should the latter be acceptable (i.e. false positives do not have serious consequences), series interpretation may be the preferred method for combining the results of these two tests. Note that these combined values assume that the tests are conditionally independent of each other. In reality, there will usually be some dependence, and then the expected values below are likely to be over-estimates of sensitivity and specificity. See Dohoo *et al.* (2009) for a more detailed discussion of this issue.

Screening and confirmatory testing

A strategy of screening and confirmatory testing is a variation on series testing and is often applied in a disease control programme. With this approach, the screening test is applied to every animal in the population to search for test-positives to which the confirmatory test is then applied. The screening test should be technically easy to apply and have a low cost. It has to be a highly sensitive test producing a high negative predictive value, since every animal negative on this test will be considered a definite negative. Its specificity should also be reasonable, so that the number of false positives that have to be subjected to the confirmatory test remains economically justifiable. The confirmatory test may require more technical expertise and more sophisticated equipment, and may be more expensive, because it is only applied to the reduced number of screening positive samples. But it has to be highly specific, and any positive reaction to the confirmatory test is considered a definitive positive. The screening and confirmatory testing approach has been applied very successfully in bovine brucellosis eradication campaigns around the world, where the Rose Bengal test was used for screening and the complement fixation test for confirmation.

Using the same test multiple times

The same test can be used in several related animals at the same time (*aggregate testing*), in animals from the same aggregate (e.g. herd) at different times (*negative-herd retesting*) or in the same animal at different times (*sequential testing*). The first and second approaches are particularly important in disease control programmes, whereas sequential testing may be used as part of research programmes, for example.

Aggregate testing

Most animal disease control programmes rely on testing of aggregate populations, in particular herds. The success of such programmes will be greatly influenced by the performance of these tests when interpreted at the herd level. It is important to recognise that with animal disease control programmes there are two units to be diagnosed: the herd and the individual animal within the herd. This approach takes advantage of the higher risk of spread within compared with between herds, mainly as a result of animals within the same herd having more opportunity for direct or indirect contact with each other than with animals from other herds. With aggregate testing, once at least one infected animal has been detected within a herd, specific measures are taken which are aimed at restricting the possibility of spread within the affected herd as well as to other herds that have susceptible animals. As an example, if as part of herd testing at least one animal tests positive to the tuberculin test for bovine tuberculosis in a cattle herd, in many countries no animals will be allowed to be sold from that herd until further assessments have demonstrated the absence of further infected animals. If one or more animals infected with a highly infectious disease such as foot-and-mouth disease is detected in a herd, all animals from that herd may be culled as a precautionary measure, even though they may have reacted negative to the test.

Many disease control programmes have been able to eradicate disease despite the relevant diagnostic tests not being highly sensitive and specific. Both bovine brucellosis and tuberculosis are examples of this. Even tests with moderate sensitivity at the individual animal level can be used because of the aggregate-level interpretation of the test. Test results from individual animals within the herds are interpreted in parallel, resulting in an increase in sensitivity at the aggregate level (= herd sensitivity), whereas aggregate-level specificity (= herd specificity) will decrease. Normally, detection of at least one positive animal will result in the herd being classified as positive. But there are some diseases where the presence of positive animals up to a certain number may still be classified as negative, since test specificity below 100% will otherwise result in too many non-infected herds being classified as positives.

Herd sensitivity and specificity are influenced by the sensitivity and specificity of individual tests, true animal level prevalence, the threshold number of test positives for classifying the herd as positive, and the number of animals tested. Herd size has a significant influence on the probability of identifying infected herds. The more animals are tested in a herd, the more likely it is to detect true positives as well as false positives. Assuming that an infected herd has at least one animal with disease, herd sensitivity quantifies the probability that a test is capable of detecting at least one of the diseased animals. This depends not only on sensitivity, but also on specificity since the infected herd may be correctly classified through individual animals being classified as false positives. Therefore, the calculation for herd sensitivity is based on apparent prevalence and the number of animals tested (see Equations 8.19 and 8.20). Herd specificity, on the other hand, only relates to non-diseased herds, and therefore is only influenced by test specificity and the number of animals tested (see Equation 8.21). The equations shown here only apply to a threshold number of at least one animal testing positive for a herd to be classified as positive. Dohoo *et al.* (2009) provides calculations for herd-level testing when threshold numbers larger than one are used.

$$Prev_{apparent} = Prev_{true} \times Se + (1 - Prev_{true}) \times (1 - Sp) \quad (8.19)$$

$$HSe = 1 - (1 - Prev_{apparent})^n \quad (8.20)$$

$$HSp = Sp^n \quad (8.21)$$

where *HSe* is herd sensitivity, *HSp* is herd specificity, $Prev_{apparent}$ is the apparent prevalence, $Prev_{true}$ is the true prevalence, *Sp* is the animal-level test specificity, *Se* is the animal-level test sensitivity and *n* is the number of animals tested.

When disease control programmes commence, prevalence of infected herds is often more than 20%. At this stage, the apparent prevalence will be higher than the true prevalence, as a consequence of less than 100% specificity of the diagnostic method. The lower the prevalence becomes, the larger the gap will be between apparent and true prevalence. Therefore, the predictive value of positive test results (at both individual animal and aggregate level) will decrease and the proportion of false positives will increase. During the early phase of a control programme, sensitivity is more important than specificity in order to ensure that all infected animals within infected herds are detected. During this phase, there will also be a larger number of herds with high prevalence compared with the later phases of the control programme. As the prevalence decreases, specificity becomes as important as sensitivity, and it may become necessary for a second test to be carried out using screening/confirmatory testing series interpretation to further increase specificity. Sensitivity is still important during this phase, since control programmes cannot afford missing too many infected animals.

Negative-herd retesting

Negative-herd retesting is an extension of the concepts described above for aggregate testing, in that the same aggregate is repeatedly tested over time. It is a testing strategy typically applied in disease control programmes. The basic principle is that only animals that were negative at the previous aggregate testing event undergo a test in the next testing event, because all animals positive at the previous test should have been removed from the herd. Interpretation of results is usually at the herd level. The testing strategy increases the chance of finding infection missed at previous aggregate testing events. In principle, the herd is asked to 'prove' that it is free from the condition. With decreasing prevalence in the population, specificity becomes more important. For example, a test with 80% specificity will produce about 20% test-positive animals in a disease-free herd.

Sequential testing

Sequential testing is used as part of specific studies where there is the opportunity to repeatedly test the same animal over time to detect seroconversion. This technique is quite powerful, as it does not have to rely on a single result for interpretation; instead, the focus can be on a significant change in test value which may well remain below a cut-off and therefore would otherwise be classified as non-diseased on the basis of single samples. Note that the repeat testing performed with this approach also means that the chance of false-positive results increases. Sequential testing can be used during experimental infection studies, for example.

Using multiple tests for different disease problems in a single animal

Batteries of multiple tests have become quite common in small animal practice, where a blood sample from a single animal is sent to a laboratory for assessment of different blood metabolite levels. The objective is to identify normal and abnormal parameters for any of these metabolites. The technique becomes useful if a set of different metabolite parameters is of diagnostic value for establishing a pattern that is considered indicative of a particular disease. The approach becomes questionable, however, if it is part of a 'fishing expedition' for a diagnosis. The clinician has to keep in mind that a cut-off for a single test is often set so that it correctly diagnoses 95% of the normal population, which means it will produce 5% false positives. As an example, with a battery of 12 diagnostic tests measuring different blood parameters, each of them may have a 0.95 probability of diagnosing a 'normal' animal correctly as negative. But it also means that the overall chance of a correct negative diagnosis on all tests is $(0.95)^{12}$ amounting to a probability of 0.54. This means that there is a 46% chance that a 'normal' animal has at least one false positive result among these 12 tests.

Decision analysis

As indicated in the introduction to this chapter, diagnoses are used to inform veterinary decision-making. The decision that is made by the veterinarian in response to a diagnosis is influenced by a number of factors, including accuracy of diagnosis, animal welfare, costs, prognosis, etc. In addition there is almost always uncertainty about the outcome of a decision, so that the decision-maker is in fact forced to gamble. In the case of veterinarians working in general practice, the uncertainty may be caused by errors in clinical and lab data, ambiguity in clinical data and variations in interpretation, uncertainty about relationships between clinical information and presence of disease, uncertainty about effects and costs of treatment and uncertainty about efficacy of control procedures and medication. Other areas where decision problems are particularly complex include the planning of disease control policies. In this situation, uncertainty is introduced, for example, through incomplete knowledge of the epidemiology of diseases or stochastic effects influencing disease spread. It is also not possible to predict the behaviour of individuals who are involved in handling and managing the disease vector or host.

Decision analysis can be applied to the decision problems described above. The process of decision analysis involves identifying all possible choices, all possible outcomes and structuring the components of the decision process in a logical and temporal sequence. *Decision tree analysis* uses a tree structure to present the different decision options and possible outcomes. The tree develops sequentially from base to terminal ends based on the components: *nodes*, *branches* and *outcomes*. There are three types of nodes: decision (= choice) nodes, chance (= probability) nodes and terminal nodes. The branches indicate the different choices if they are extending from a decision node and the different outcomes if they are extending from a chance node. Each of the branches emanating from a chance node has associated probabilities and each of the terminal ends has an associated utility or value. In the case of decision trees a solution is typically obtained through choosing the alternative with the highest expected monetary value. This is calculated through folding back the tree. Starting from the terminal nodes and moving back to the root of the tree, expected values are calculated at each chance node as the weighted average of possible outcomes where the weights are the chances of particular outcome occurrences. At each decision node the branch with the highest expected value is chosen as the preferred alternative. Decision tree analysis has the advantage that it encourages one to break down complex problems into simpler components such as choices, probabilistic events and alternative outcomes. It requires the weighting of risks and benefits and the logical sequencing of components, as well as explicit estimates of probabilities. Concern about utilities is encouraged by the need to place values on them. Critical determinants of the decision problem can be identified and areas of insufficient knowledge can be indicated.

As an example of a veterinary decision problem, a client has to decide whether to rest a horse valued at $5000 diagnosed with lameness, without incurring any additional expenditure, or to spend $500 on surgery. The

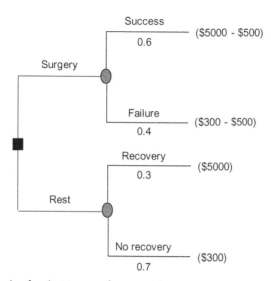

Figure 8.8   Example of a decision tree for equine lameness treatment.

decision tree is shown in Figure 8.8. The assumptions being made are that the probability of recovery is 0.6 for surgery and 0.3 for rest. The salvage value for the horse would be $300. The expected monetary values for the two treatments are calculated as follows:

- expected value for surgery:

$$EV_{surgery} = 0.6 \times (\$5000 - \$500) + 0.4 \times (\$300 - \$500) = \$2620$$

- expected value for rest:

$$EV_{rest} = 0.3 \times \$5000 + 0.7 \times \$300 = \$1710$$

The interpretation of these results is that in the long run the surgery is more profitable, assuming that the values and probabilities are chosen correctly. Further examples of decision analysis applications in animal health can be found in Slenning (2001) and Smith (2006).

Informing disease control and eradication

Learning objectives

After completing this chapter, you will be able to:

- Describe the principles of risk analysis.
- Understand the principles of herd health and productivity assessment.
- Provide an overview of animal health surveillance methods.
- Describe the steps involved in outbreak investigation.
- Discuss the issues associated with modelling of animal health data.
- List various applications of computerised information technology in animal health.

Introduction

Epidemiology has made a major contribution to veterinary science particularly in the area of integrating science-based methodologies into veterinary decision-making, thereby contributing towards an enhanced objectivity of the process. One of the key elements has been the introduction of risk and uncertainty concepts into animal health. These can be applied formally under the risk analysis framework for a wide range of veterinary activities, covering the whole spectrum from individual animal and herd to national and international disease management. Many advances have been made in this area over the last 20 years, and the access to fast, networked and relatively low-cost electronic data entry, storage and retrieval systems has been instrumental to these developments. An important deficiency remains the variation in data quality, which has not improved at the same pace as data quantity. As a result, the degree of uncertainty associated with the outputs generated by these systems has not necessarily diminished, and in some aspects has even increased. One of the challenges for epidemiologists working with such information systems is to communicate these uncertainties to end users, whether they are owners of pets or farm animals, or decision-makers in relation to national and international disease control policies.

Data collection to inform risk analysis can be conducted at different levels of aggregation. At the herd level, farmers collect data to be able to optimise animal health, welfare and productivity. National animal disease surveillance programmes involve data collection that is used to inform risk assessment and management for the purpose of improving or maintaining the health and welfare status of a national or regional animal population. Any such data collection system needs to be linked to analytical tools that allow extraction of important patterns with respect to animal health, welfare or productivity, and potential associated risk factors. This will include the use of various types of models which may be used to explain or predict patterns of disease, welfare and productivity. Epidemiological principles are an integral part of these applications, in particular in relation to representativeness, bias and interpretation of cause–effect relationships.

Risk analysis

The recognition of the relevance of adopting the risk analysis framework in the context of animal health decision-making has had a significant impact in particular on veterinary services at the national level. But the approach is also applicable to other types of epidemiological units, such as individual animals or herds, as well as for human food. Risk analysis is defined as a structured, science-based and transparent approach to risk management. It involves estimation of the risk of adverse events and their mitigation. The World Organisation for Animal Health (OIE) has included risk analysis into the Terrestrial Animal Health Code for the purpose of managing risks resulting from imports of animals and their products (Vallat 2008), but the methodology applies to any situation involving management of the risk of introduction and spread of an infectious disease. Figure 9.1 shows the components of risk analysis, as defined in the OIE's Terrestrial Animal Health Code (Vallat 2008), the main ones being hazard identification, risk assessment, risk management and risk communication.

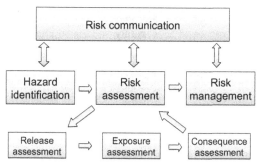

Figure 9.1   Risk analysis framework.*

Hazard identification is the process of defining the infectious organism that could be introduced to the epidemiological unit of interest, e.g. animal, herd, region or country. Once this has been done, a *risk assessment* needs to be conducted. This is the process of defining risk(s) associated with the hazard. It begins with defining a precise risk question, such as 'What is the risk per year of introducing *Mycobacterium bovis* infection into dairy cattle herds in south-west England?' The next step is the development of a risk pathway diagram where all mechanisms relevant to the introduction of the hazard are represented. This part of the process will also identify any gaps in relation to the epidemiology of the hazard. The development of the risk assessment model can be done using qualitative or quantitative methods. Qualitative methods are usually used when few quantitative data are available. The risk assessment is structured into three components (see Figure 9.2). The first is the *release assessment* which deals with the introduction of the hazard to the epidemiological unit of interest. The second, the *exposure assessment*, addresses the likelihood of susceptible animals becoming exposed to the hazard, given that it has been released. The third component is the *consequence assessment*, which is about the likelihood of infection and further spread, given exposure.

Figure 9.3 shows an example of the structure of a risk release assessment model, which has been kept very simple for the purpose of introducing the basic concepts of risk assessment models. The risk question in this case could be: 'What is the probability that at least one chicken infected with disease X is imported into country Y per month?' It starts with the expected number of chickens imported during 1 month. The probability of an animal being infected and not detected by the diagnostic test is calculated using the product between

---

* This illustration is inspired by two figures published in the OIE (World Organisation for Animal Health) *Terrestrial Animal Health Code* (http://www.oie.int/eng/normes/en_mcode. htm?e1d10), 2008, Seventeenth Edition (Fig. 1: The four components of risk analysis, on page 25, Chapter 2.1, article 2.1.1; and Fig. 1: Import risk analysis, on page 27, Chapter 2.2, article 2.2.1).

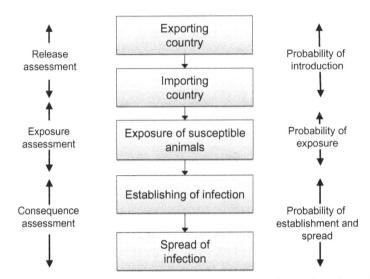

Figure 9.2   Components of a risk assessment model for import of animals or derived products.

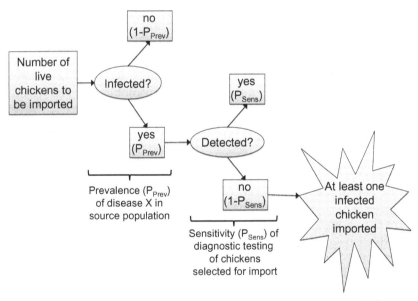

Figure 9.3   Example of the structure of a quantitative release assessment model for the risk of importation of chickens infected with disease X into country Y.

prevalence (P_{Prev}) and the probability of a false negative ($1 - P_{Sens}$). One minus that probability gives the chance that this does not happen to a random animal ($1 - P_{Prev}(1 - P_{Sens})$) among those imported. The question is now how likely it is that the latter happens to all animals that will be imported during the month. This is calculated by exponentiating the probability of no animal being a false negative with the total number of animals n to be imported: $(1 - P_{\text{Prev}}(1 - P_{\text{Sens}}))^n$. Subtracting the resulting probability from 1 gives the probability that at least one infected animal will be imported during that month. Using $n = 1000$ for the number of chickens to be imported in the month, a disease prevalence of $P_{\text{Prev}} = 0.1$ and a test sensitivity of $P_{\text{Sens}} = 0.99$, there is a 63% probability that at least one infected chicken will be imported in the month:

$$p = 1 - (1 - 0.1(1 - 0.99))^{1000} = 0.63$$

The mathematical basis for the above formula is discussed in detail in Vose (2008).

The results of the risk assessment are used to decide on appropriate *risk management*, which is the process of formulating and implementing measures designed to reduce the likelihood of the unwanted event occurring or the magnitude of its consequences. At this stage of the process, risks have to be balanced against the benefits, and results from economic analyses will often have to be considered. It is important to have effective risk communication throughout the risk analysis process in place. This includes communication between all important stakeholders, i.e. decision-makers in relation to animal health such as farmers and government officials, as well as scientists and in many circumstances the general public. Effective risk communication will contribute to the transparency of the risk analysis, and thereby facilitate its acceptance by key stakeholders. There are now many examples of risk assessment applications relating to animal health (e.g. Pfeiffer *et al.* 2006; Hartnett *et al.* 2007). More detail on the risk analysis approach can be found in Vose (2008), Anonymous (2004a) and Anonymous (2004b).

Assessment of herd health and productivity

Traditionally, animal disease control mainly focused on monitoring of disease outbreaks and movements of disease agents. In recent times, many livestock farmers have recognised the need to continuously collect herd data for setting priorities and defining actions aimed at improving animal health, welfare and productivity. Computerised record-keeping has been used particularly in intensive pig and dairy production for over 20 years. One of the advantages of these information systems is that farmers can generate quantitative production performance parameters, such as shown in Figure 9.4 for reproductive performance on pig farms. The top-level parameter in this diagnostic indicator tree, pigs weaned per sow per year, should be continuously monitored and compared with retrospective data from the same herd or the distribution of values in similar farms. If the number of pigs weaned per sow per year is considered to be too low as a result of that comparison, then the parameters further down in the flowchart, i.e. litter size and litters per sow per year, should be compared

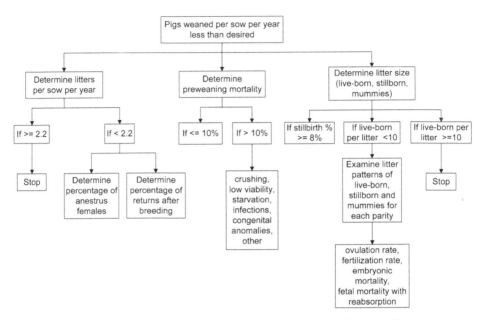

Figure 9.4 Flowchart of diagnostic indicator tree for poor reproductive performance in pig production (adapted from Straw *et al.* 2006). Reproduced with permission from Wiley-Blackwell.

with benchmark figures. Continuing this process towards the relevant terminal ends of the tree should allow identifying the potential causes of the performance problem, and therefore inform targeted use of further diagnostic tools or even immediate treatment action. The integration of epidemiological principles into management of livestock health and production is presented in more detail in Radostits (2001).

Disease surveillance and monitoring

Both disease surveillance and monitoring imply a process of regular data collection. Monitoring is a more general term, referring to a continuous data collection effort for detecting changes or trends in the occurrence of an event of interest. Surveillance, on the hand, implies systematic collection, analysis and interpretation of animal health-related events occurring in a population, and should include a tailored data collection and analysis system, predefined thresholds in relation to disease occurrence and predefined interventions subject to results obtained from the surveillance system. Its objective is to meet basic information needs in order to assess and manage risks effectively, i.e. to minimise, as far as practicable, taking into account costs and benefits, the probability of adverse effects occurring on public health, trade in animals and animal products, and animal health and welfare (Anonymous 2000). It is aimed at detection and early warning in relation to new and emerging disease as well as disease vectors. Monitoring of endemic disease and its vectors is conducted with the aim of characterising changes in disease occurrence levels, their relative ranking and importance, and assessing the impact of control programmes. The data collected through a surveillance system need to be processed and analysed, and the results should be used to inform risk assessment and management. Considering these aims, a surveillance system is usually structured into separate programmes each of which deals with one specific outcome, such as determining the level of a particular endemic disease. A surveillance system also consists of several data collection components, such as government and private laboratory services, border inspection and slaughterhouse inspection as well as specific disease testing programme. Each of these will make particular contributions to specific surveillance programmes. It is useful to characterise individual components within surveillance programmes using the following set of criteria: objectives, hazard definition, case definition, unit of interest, diagnostic methods, target population, location, timing, data collection and processing, data analysis, communication and dissemination of results.

Based on the data collection method, surveillance system components can be grouped into passive or active surveillance activities. *Passive surveillance* includes laboratory submission and case reporting by the public. It also includes *molecular surveillance* where diagnoses of specific infectious organisms are further differentiated into molecular strains. These data on genetic relatedness can then be used to develop hypotheses about sources of infection. *Active surveillance* refers to data collection based on structured population sampling supported by a clearly defined objective. It includes disease prevalence surveys, risk-based and sentinel surveillance. *Risk-based surveillance* employs epidemiological and economic principles to define the activities within a surveillance programme (Stärk *et al.* 2006). *Sentinel surveillance* involves continuous monitoring of herds, usually selected based on risk, to be able to detect outbreaks of disease or introductions of infection as early as possible. This type of surveillance is particularly useful for monitoring the occurrence of vector-borne diseases (Racloz *et al.* 2006). More recently, the concept of *syndromic surveillance* has been introduced, in the first instance as a tool for early warning against bioterrorism attacks. It uses various non-specific diagnostic indicators, such as a sudden reduction in reproductive performance in livestock, to warn of outbreaks of diseases. A problem with this approach is that it has a low specificity, and therefore may result in too many false alarms. The ability of surveillance programme components to detect a particular disease can be quantified as surveillance sensitivity and specificity using scenario-tree analysis (Hadorn and Stark 2008; Martin *et al.* 2007). Further details about surveillance systems can be found in Thrusfield (2005) and Salman (2003).

In developing countries, it is often impossible to conduct animal disease surveillance of a high standard using the costly methods applied in developed countries. In many such countries, the introduction of community animal health care services will allow some level of disease surveillance. In such systems, so-called 'barefoot' veterinarians provide the most common animal health services to farmers; these services in turn may have been defined using epidemiological surveys, longitudinal studies or herd health and productivity profiling. Data quality is often influenced by a lack of stakeholder commitment towards the aims of the data collection and analysis. In such circumstances, participatory rural appraisal methods can be used to collect data (Jost *et al.* 2007; Loader and Amartya 1999). This methodology has as a particular focus on the establishment of trust among the farmers by identifying and recognising their priorities and needs. The approach should result in more accurate data, although because of the lack of a statistical sampling framework it can be more difficult to analyse and draw generalisable inferences.

Outbreak investigation

As described earlier, an outbreak is a series of disease events clustered in time, which is usually detected by one of the components of a surveillance system, such as farmer reporting. An outbreak investigation may be conducted in response to the detection of an outbreak. The aim is to understand the cause, to identify methods for controlling it and to prevent any future occurrences. It is important to recognise that outbreak investigations for diseases with high animal and public health impact should be conducted by multidisciplinary teams, involving clinical, laboratory, epidemiological and other relevant expertise.

The following steps could be taken during an outbreak investigation:

1. Confirm the existence of an outbreak.
2. Establish a diagnosis:
   - Generate a definitive or tentative diagnosis, followed by a detailed clinico-pathological assessment.
   - Produce a case definition that is as specific as possible, excluding possible differential diagnoses.
   - Identify molecular strain characteristics (where applicable).
3. Determine the magnitude of the problem (i.e. quantify risk):
   - Count cases.
   - Establish population at risk (i.e. denominator).
   - Compute the incidence risk and compare it with normal or expected risks of disease.

4. Analyse the problem in terms of when, where and who:
    *   Analyse the *temporal pattern* (= when) by constructing an epidemic curve, and attempt to estimate incubation and exposure periods.
    *   Analyse the *spatial pattern* (= where), e.g. by drawing a sketch map of the area or the layout of the affected farm or farm building(s). The investigator should inspect the drawing for possible interrelationships among cases, and between location and cases and other physical features.
    *   Analyse the *animal pattern* (= who), e.g. by investigating factors such as age, sex and breed. This may involve quantitative analysis by calculating risk ratios and particularly risk differences, testing of any associations between disease and risk factors for statistical significance as well as potentially conducting multivariable analyses to determine which risk factors are most important. This will lead to a list of potentially causal factors associated with the disease.
5. Develop working hypothesis:
    Based on the findings in the data analysis conducted under step 4, a working hypothesis should be developed with respect to potential causes, sources, mode of transmission and exposure period.
6. Evaluate working hypothesis:
    If possible, the working hypothesis should be tested using an experimental study.
7. Further data collection and analyses:
    *   Conduct detailed follow-up investigations:
        With complex problems not revealing any quick answers with respect to the source of the problem, it is often advisable to conduct an intensive follow-up. This would involve a clinical, pathological, microbiological and toxicological examination of tissues, feeds, objects, etc. Detailed diagrams of feed preparation or movement of animals could be prepared and a search for additional cases on other premises or outbreaks of similar nature in other locations could be conducted. This will also include a review of the published literature.
    *   Perform an economic analysis:
        Possible interventions should be evaluated based on cost-benefit or cost-effectiveness analyses.
8. Communicate findings:
    *   The outcome of the outbreak investigation should be presented as a written report containing recommendations for controlling the outbreak and preventing further occurrences.

Published examples of outbreak investigations are Thurmond (1986), Wilesmith *et al.* (1988), Yeruham *et al.* (2003) and Irvine *et al.* (2007). Waldner

(2001) presents a detailed introduction to outbreak investigation for herd health problems.

Modelling

Investigations aimed at understanding epidemiological systems often involve the development of a model of the system. Models are needed where mental simulation is not able to represent multiple causal links within a system (Lempert *et al.* 2003). According to Klein (1998), the limit is usually reached with three key variables and six transitions from one state to another. Models can be very simple or complex, and they can be conceptual diagrammatic representations of the biological relationships or allow dynamic simulations of the system. The statistical analysis of epidemiological data often involves the development of *data-driven models*. They involve expressing the relationship between various risk factors and an outcome variable, typically using a linear equation with a statistical algorithm determining each risk factor's weighting. With *knowledge-driven models*, the researcher specifies the risk factors and their parameter values, based on epidemiological understanding and existing data. These include the risk assessment models described above, as well as *mathematical* and *simulation models*. Knowledge-driven models can be static or dynamic. *Dynamic models* are used to represent dynamic processes or systems and simulate their behaviour through time. They mimic the system under study which allows testing of specific hypotheses, e.g. about the epidemiology of an infectious process, such as the likely impact of control measures or to identify gaps in our understanding which need further investigation. Figure 9.5 shows an example of how a model might represent the dynamics of disease pathogenesis in an individual animal. The transitions between different states of the animal in relation to the pathogenetic process can be modelled using probabilities. For the model to be able to represent the dynamics within a population, it is also necessary to represent mechanisms for transmission. This will then lead to a transmission pattern such as shown in Figure 9.6, where each infected animal has a chance of infecting other susceptible animals within the in-contact population. A commonly used approach to dynamic modelling is to represent a population as a series of compartments, e.g. susceptible, infected and recovered/immune compartments, and to then use differential equations for expressing the rate of flow of animals between compartments. This approach is also called *SIR (susceptible/infectious/recovered) modelling*. One important output parameter from such models is the basic reproductive ratio R_0 (also basic reproductive number, basic reproductive rate) which quantifies the average number of animals becoming infected per infectious animal in a susceptible population (Heffernan *et al.* 2005). It is influenced by the duration of infectiousness, the number

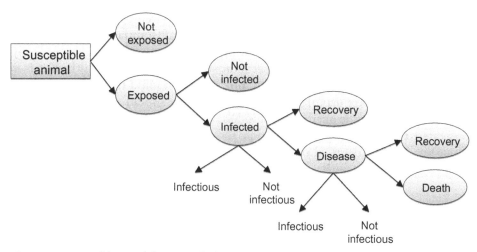

Figure 9.5   Possible states of an animal relevant to dynamic epidemiological modelling in relation to the pathogenesis of an infectious disease.

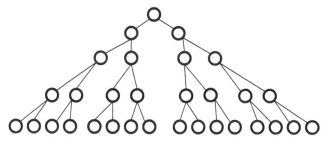

Figure 9.6   Spread of infection through a population (grey, infected; white, non-infected).

of contacts and the probability of transmission. $R_0 > 1$ means that an infection continues to spread. Such models can then be used to identify control strategies that reduce R_0 below 1, and therefore result in stopping the spread of infection.

As part of a decision support system, models can be used to test alternative strategies. The tools used for the development of such models include computerised spreadsheets that allow non-programmers to construct simple models. Computer programming languages have to be used in developing more complex models. Before any models or their outputs are used to inform the decision-making process, they need to be validated. This is much less controversial for data-driven models than it is for knowledge-driven models. The main reason for this is that the former are based on more or less objectively collected data, and assuming that the data were collected without major bias their internal and external validity can be described in quantitative terms. Because knowledge-driven models are to a significant extent a reflection of the hypotheses about the system relationships made by the model developers, their validity is difficult to assess and therefore often provides substantial opportunity for controversy (Kitching *et al.* 2006). Undoubtedly models will increasingly become an important element of decision support in animal health. But it is useful to keep the statement made by Box (1979) in mind that 'all models are wrong, but some are useful'. Potential model users should not expect it to be necessary to prove the accuracy of models, but rather that it needs to be demonstrated that they are good enough for the intended purpose. Thrusfield (2005) provides a detailed overview of dynamic modelling approaches in the context of animal health.

Computerised information systems

The explosion in the amount of information that we need to handle on a day-to-day basis has resulted in the need to develop more efficient means of information management. Various types of computerised information systems have been developed which allow the input, storage, retrieval and analysis of various types of data. The data may be collected by a farmer on production animal performance or health, by a veterinary practitioner about client case histories, or by laboratories in relation to disease diagnoses. It can also include scientific information, such as peer-reviewed publications. Such an information system may operate on a single computer, be networked locally or be accessible through the internet.

The internet has become a key mechanism for information access. There are various general search engines, such as Google, which facilitate access to all information publicly accessible available on the internet. A major criticism is the lack of a quality check when using this type of search. Although end users now have access to much more information, they need to take on a more active role in determining what is good information and what not. *Wikipedia* is a free electronic encyclopedia where everybody can edit content, and a specialised veterinary online knowledge base has been developed by UK veterinary schools (www.wikivet.net). The electronic edition of the *Merck Veterinary Manual* (see www.merckvetmanual.com) is an example of a textbook that is now also published via the internet. The most up-to-date scientific literature can be searched through bibliographic access systems such as PubMed (www.pubmed.gov), and full text publications can be accessed via open access publishers' websites such as BioMed Central (www.biomedcentral. com) as well as several paid access sites.

The information systems presented above are solely aimed at information retrieval, not analysis. To assist veterinarians in making diagnoses, artificial intelligence methods including knowledge-based systems (expert systems) or neural networks can be used. Examples of such systems are BOVID and

CANID, which are probabilistic expert systems used for diagnoses of cattle and canine disease problems respectively. Herd health management increasingly involves the use of computerised recording and monitoring systems such as PigWIN. Modern national disease control programmes have computerised database management systems as an essential component. The RADAR system developed in the United Kingdom combines different data sources which can be accessed by various types of users, and it also runs a range of analyses (Paiba *et al.* 2007). A significant problem that these systems have to deal with is the variation in data quality, and how to communicate this to the end user. This is probably one reason why the vision developed over the last 5–10 years of computerised decision support systems that integrate databases, expert systems and simulation models has not quite become reality yet (Morris *et al.* 2002).

References

Altman, D.G., Machin, D., Bryant, T.N. and Gardner, M.J. (2000) *Statistics with Confidence*. BMJ Books, London.

Anderson, I. (2002) *Foot and Mouth Disease 2001: Lessons to be learned inquiry report*. The Stationery Office, London.

Anderson, R.M., Fraser, C., Ghani, A.C., *et al.* (2004) Epidemiology, transmission dynamics and control of SARS: the 2002–2003 epidemic. *Philosophical Transactions of the Royal Society of London Series B, Biological Sciences*, **359**, 1091–105.

Anonymous (2000) *Veterinary Surveillance in England and Wales – A Review*. Ministry of Agriculture, Fisheries and Food, London.

Anonymous (2004a) *Handbook on Import Risk Analysis for Animals and Animal Products: Introduction and Qualitative Risk Analysis*. OIE Publications, Paris.

Anonymous (2004b) *Handbook on Import Risk Analysis for Animals and Animal Products: Quantitative Risk Analysis*. OIE Publications, Paris.

Anonymous (2006) *Bluetongue Serotype 8 Epidemic Bulletin – Outbreak Period until 30 October 2006*. European Food Safety Authority, Parma.

Box, G.E.P. (1979) Robustness in the strategy of scientific model building. In: *Robustness in Statistics* (eds R.L Launer and G.N. Wilkinson). Academic Press, New York.

Caswell, J.L. and Archambault, M. (2007) *Mycoplasma bovis* pneumonia in cattle. *Animal Health Research Reviews*, **8**, 161–86.

Cockcroft, P. and Holmes, M. (2003) *Handbook of Evidence-Based Veterinary Medicine*. Blackwell Publishing, Oxford.

Dabo, S.M., Taylor, J.D. and Confer, A.W. (2007) *Pasteurella multocida* and bovine respiratory disease. *Animal Health Research Reviews*, 8, 129–50.

Defra (2009) *Bovine tuberculosis in England: towards eradication*. Defra, London.

Dohoo, I.R., Martin, W. and Stryhn, H. (2009) *Veterinary Epidemiologic Research*. AVC Inc., Charlottetown, Prince Edward Island, Canada.

Evans, A.S. (1976) Causation and disease: the Henle-Koch postulates revisited. *Yale Journal of Biology and Medicine*, 49, 175–95.

Falkow, S. (2004) Molecular Koch's postulates applied to bacterial pathogenicity – a personal recollection 15 years later. *Nature Reviews Microbiology*, 2, 67–72.

Fletcher, R.W. and Fletcher, S.W. (2005) *Clinical Epidemiology: The Essentials*. Lippincott Williams & Wilkins, Philadelphia.

Fredericks, D.N. and Relman, D.A. (1996) Sequence-based identification of microbial pathogens: a reconsideration of Koch's postulates. *Clinical Microbiology Reviews*, 9, 18–33.

Gibbens, J.C. and Wilesmith, J.W. (2002) Temporal and geographical distribution of cases of foot-and-mouth disease during the early weeks of the 2001 epidemic in Great Britain. *Veterinary Record*, 151, 407–12.

Greenhalgh, T. (2006) *How to Read A Paper – The Basics of Evidence-Based Medicine*. BMJ Books, London.

Greiner, M., Pfeiffer, D. and Smith, R.D. (2000) Principles and practical application of the receiver-operating characteristic analysis for diagnostic tests. *Preventive Veterinary Medicine*, 45, 23–41.

Gross, R. (1999) *Making Medical Decisions*. American College of Physicians, Philadelphia.

Hadorn, D.C. and Stark, K.D. (2008) Evaluation and optimization of surveillance systems for rare and emerging infectious diseases. *Veterinary Research*, 39, 57.

Hartnett, E., Adkin, A., Seaman, M., *et al*. (2007) A quantitative assessment of the risks from illegally imported meat contaminated with foot and mouth disease virus to Great Britain. *Risk Analysis*, 27, 187–202.

Heffernan, J.M., Smith, R.J. and Wahl, L.M. (2005) Perspectives on the basic reproductive ratio. *Journal of The Royal Society Interface*, 2, 281–93.

Hill, A.B. (1965) The environment and disease: association or causation? *Proceedings of the Royal Society of Medicine*, **58**, 295–300.

Houe, H., Ersboll, A.K. and Toft, N. (2004) *Introduction to Veterinary Epidemiology*. Biofolia, Frederiksberg, Denmark.

Humphry, R.W., Cameron, A. and Gunn, G.J. (2004) A practical approach to calculate sample size for herd prevalence surveys. *Preventive Veterinary Medicine*, **65**, 173–88.

Irvine, R.M., Banks, J., Londt, B.Z., *et al.* (2007) Outbreak of highly pathogenic avian influenza caused by Asian lineage H5N1 virus in turkeys in Great Britain in January 2007. *Veterinary Record*, **161**, 100–1.

Jordan, D. and McEwen, S.A. (1998) Herd-level test performance based on uncertain estimates of individual test performance, individual true prevalence and herd true prevalence. *Preventive Veterinary Medicine*, **36**, 187–209.

Jost, C.C., Mariner, J.C., Roeder, P.L., Sawitri, E. and Macgregor-Skinner, G.J. (2007) Participatory epidemiology in disease surveillance and research. *Revue Scientifique et Technique – Office International des Epizooties*, **26**, 537–49.

Khoury, M.J., Millikan, R. and Gwinn, M. (2008) Genetic and molecular epidemiology. In: *Modern Epidemiology* (eds K.J. Rothman, S. Greenland and T.L. Lash), pp. 564–79. Lippincott Williams & Wilkins, Philadelphia.

Kitching, R.P., Thrusfield, M.V. and Taylor, N.M. (2006) Use and abuse of mathematical models: an illustration from the 2001 foot and mouth disease epidemic in the United Kingdom. *Revue Scientifique et Technique – Office International des Epizooties*, **25**, 293–311.

Klein, G. (1998) *Sources of Power: How People Make Decisions*. MIT Press, Cambridge, MA.

Kraemer, H.C. (1992) *Evaluating Medical Tests – Objective and Quantitative Guidelines*. Sage Publications, Newbury Park, CA.

Lempert, R.J., Popper, S.W. and Bankes, S.C. (2003) *Shaping the Next One Hundred Years – New Methods for Quantitative, Long-Term Policy Analysis*. RAND Corporation, Santa Monica, CA.

Levy, P.S. and Lemeshow, S. (2008) *Sampling of Populations: Methods and Applications*. John Wiley & Sons, New York.

Lipkin, W.I. (2008) Pathogen discovery. *PLoS Pathogens*, **4**, e1000002.

Loader, R. and Amartya, L. (1999) Participatory rural appraisal: extending the research methods base. *Agricultural Systems*, **62**, 73–85.

Mackintosh, C.G., Schollum, L.M., Harris, R.E. *et al.* (1980) Epidemiology of leptospirosis in dairy farm workers in the Manawatu: Part I: A cross-sectional serological survey and associated occupational factors. *New Zealand Veterinary Journal*, **28**, 245–50.

Martin, P.A., Cameron, A.R. and Greiner, M. (2007) Demonstrating freedom from disease using multiple complex data sources 1: a new methodology based on scenario trees. *Preventive Veterinary Medicine*, **79**, 71–97.

Morris, J.A. and Gardner, M.J. (2000) Epidemiological studies. In: *Statistics with Confidence* (eds D.G. Altman, D. Machin, T.N. Bryant and M.J. Gardner), pp. 57–72. BMJ Books, London.

Morris, R.S., Sanson, R.L., Stern, M.W., Stevenson, M. and Wilesmith, J.W. (2002) Decision-support tools for foot and mouth disease control. *Revue Scientifique et Technique – Office International des Epizooties*, **21**, 557–67.

Nielsen, S.S., Houe, H., Ersbøll, A.K. and Toft, N. (2004) Evaluating diagnostic tests. In: *Introduction to Veterinary Epidemiology* (eds H. Houe, A.K. Ersbøll and N. Toft), pp. 133–51. Biofolia, Frederiksberg, Denmark.

Noordhuizen, J.P.T.M., Thrusfield, M.V., Frankena, K. and Graat, E.A.M. (2001) *Application of Quantitative Methods in Veterinary Epidemiology*. Wageningen Pers, Wageningen.

Page, G.P., George, V., Go, R.C., Page, P.Z. and Allison, D.B. (2003) 'Are we there yet?': Deciding when one has demonstrated specific genetic causation in complex diseases and quantitative traits. *American Journal of Human Genetics*, **73**, 711–19.

Paiba, G.A., Roberts, S.R., Houston, C.W. *et al.* (2007) UK surveillance: provision of quality assured information from combined datasets. *Preventive Veterinary Medicine*, **81**, 117–34.

Pfeiffer, D.U. (2008) Animal tuberculosis. In: *Clinical Tuberculosis* (eds P.D.O. Davies, P.F. Barnes and S.B. Gordon), pp. 519–28. Hodder Arnold, London.

Pfeiffer, D.U., Brown, I., Fouchier, R.A.M., *et al.* (2006) Migratory birds and their possible role in the spread of highly pathogenic avian influenza. *EFSA Journal*, **357**, 1–46.

Pfeiffer, D.U., Minh, P.Q., Martin, V., Epprecht, M. and Otte, M.J. (2007) An analysis of the spatial and temporal patterns of highly pathogenic avian influenza occurrence in Vietnam using national surveillance data. *Veterinary Journal*, **174**, 8.

Racloz, V., Griot, C. and Stark, K.D. (2006) Sentinel surveillance systems with special focus on vector-borne diseases. *Animal Health Research Review*, 7, 71–9.

Radostits, O.M. (2001) *Herd Health*. W.B. Saunders, Philadelphia.

Radostits, O.M., Gay, C.C., Hinchcliff, K.W. and Constable, P.D. (2007) *Veterinary Medicine – A Textbook of the Diseases of Cattle, Sheep, Pigs, Goats and Horses*. W.B. Saunders, London.

Reichel, M.P. and Pfeiffer, D.U. (2002) An analysis of the performance characteristics of serological tests for the diagnosis of *Neospora caninum* infection in cattle. *Veterinary Parasitology*, **107**, 197–207.

Rice, J.A., Carrasco-Medina, L., Hodgins, D.C. and Shewen, P.E. (2007) *Mannheimia haemolytica* and bovine respiratory disease. *Animal Health Research Review*, 8, 117–28.

Rothman, K.J. (2002) *Epidemiology – An Introduction*. Oxford University Press, Oxford.

Rothman, K.J., Greenland, S. and Lash, T.L. (2008a) Validity in epidemiological studies. In: *Modern Epidemiology* (eds K.J. Rothman, S. Greenland and T.L. Lash), pp. 128–47. Lippincott Williams & Wilkins, Philadelphia.

Rothman, K.J., Greenland, S. and Lash, T.L. (2008b) Precision and statistics in epidemiologic studies. In: *Modern Epidemiology* (eds K.J. Rothman, S. Greenland and T.L. Lash), pp. 148–67. Lippincott Williams & Wilkins, Philadelphia.

Rothman, K.J., Greenland, S. and Lash, T.L. (2008c) Case–control studies. In: *Modern Epidemiology* (eds K.J. Rothman, S. Greenland and T.L. Lash), pp. 111–27. Lippincott Williams & Wilkins, Philadelphia.

Rothman, K.J., Greenland, S. and Lash, T.L. (2008d) *Modern Epidemiology*. Lippincott Williams & Wilkins, Philadelphia.

Rothman, K.J., Greenland, S., Poole, C., Lash, T.L. (2008e) Causation and causal inference. In: *Modern Epidemiology* (eds K.J. Rothman, S. Greenland and T.L. Lash), pp. 5–31. Lippincott Williams & Wilkins, Philadelphia.

Rushton, J. (2008) *The Economics of Animal Health and Production*. CABI, Wallingford, Oxon.

Salman, M.D. (2003) *Animal Disease Surveillance and Survey Systems: Methods and Applications*. Wiley–Blackwell, Chichester.

Slenning, B.D. (2001) Quantitative tools for production-oriented veterinarians. In: *Herd Health* (ed. O.M. Radostits), pp. 47–106. W.B. Saunders, Philadelphia.

Smith, R.D. (2006) *Veterinary Clinical Epidemiology*. CRC Press, Boca Raton, FL.

Stärk, K.D., Regula, G., Hernandez, J., *et al.* (2006) Concepts for risk-based surveillance in the field of veterinary medicine and veterinary public health: review of current approaches. *BMC Health Service Research*, **6**, 20.

Stegeman, A., Bouma, A., Elbers, A.R., *et al.* (2004) Avian influenza A virus (H7N7) epidemic in the Netherlands in 2003: course of the epidemic and effectiveness of control measures. *Journal of Infectious Diseases*, **190**, 2088–95.

Stegeman, A., Elbers, A., de, S.H., Moser, H., Smak, J. and Pluimers, F. (2000) The 1997–1998 epidemic of classical swine fever in the Netherlands. *Veterinary Microbiology*, **73**, 183–96.

Straw, B.E., Dewey, C.E. and Wilson, M.R. (2006) Differential diagnosis of disease. In: *Diseases of Swine* (eds B.E. Straw, J.J. Zimmermann, S. d'Allaire and D.J. Taylor), pp. 241–86. Blackwell Publishing, Ames, IA.

Thompson, S.K. (2002) *Sampling*. John Wiley & Sons, New York.

Thompson, S.K. and Collins, L.M. (2002) Adaptive sampling in research on risk-related behaviors. *Drug and Alcohol Dependence*, **68**, 57–67.

Thrusfield, M.V. (2005) *Veterinary Epidemiology*. Blackwell Science, Oxford.

Thurmond, M.C. (1986) Epidemiologic approaches used in a herd health practice to investigate neonatal calf mortality. *Preventive Veterinary Medicine*, **4**, 317–28.

Toma, B., Dufour, B., Sanaa, M., *et al.* (1999) *Applied Veterinary Epidemiology and the Control of Disease in Populations*. AEEMA, Maisons-Alfort.

Vallat, B. (2008) *Terrestrial Animal Health Code*. World Organisation for Animal Health, Paris.

Vose, D. (2008) *Risk Analysis – A Quantitative Guide*. John Wiley & Sons, Chichester.

Wagner, B. and Salman, M.D. (2004) Strategies for two-stage sampling designs for estimating herd-level prevalence. *Preventive Veterinary Medicine*, **66**, 1–17.

Waldner, C. (2001) Investigation of disease outbreaks and suboptimal productivity in herds. In: *Herd Health* (ed. O.M. Radostits), pp. 189–209. W.B. Saunders, Philadelphia.

Wilesmith, J.W., Ryan, J.B.M. and Atkinson, M.J. (1991) Bovine spongiform encephalopathy: epidemiological studies on the origin. *Veterinary Record*, **128**, 199–203.

Wilesmith, J.W., Wells, G.A., Cranwell, M.P. and Ryan, J.B. (1988) Bovine spongiform encephalopathy: epidemiological studies. *Veterinary Record*, **123**, 638–44.

Yeruham, I., Elad, D., Avidar, Y., Grinberg, K., Tiomkin, D. and Monbaz, A. (2003) Outbreak of botulism type B in a dairy cattle herd: clinical and epidemiological aspects. *Veterinary Record*, **153**, 270–2.

Zinsstag, J., Schelling, E., Wyss, K. and Mahamat, M.B. (2005) Potential of cooperation between human and animal health to strengthen health systems. *The Lancet*, **366**, 2142–5.

Index

Printed in the United States
By Bookmasters